Chest Wall Deformities and Corrective Procedures

Shyam K. Kolvekar • Hans K. Pilegaard
Editors

Chest Wall Deformities and Corrective Procedures

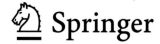

Editors
Shyam K. Kolvekar
Consultant Cardiothoracic Surgeon
The Heart Hospital UCLH
London
UK

Hans K. Pilegaard
Associate. Professor
Department of Cardiothoracic and
Vascular Surgery
Department of Clinical Medicine
Aarhus University Hospital, Denmark
Aarhus
Denmark

ISBN 978-3-319-23966-8   ISBN 978-3-319-23968-2   (eBook)
DOI 10.1007/978-3-319-23968-2

Library of Congress Control Number: 2015957217

Springer Cham Heidelberg New York Dordrecht London

Printed on acid-free paper

Springer International Publishing AG Switzerland is part of Springer Science+Business Media
(www.springer.com)

Preface

Chest wall deformities can be categorized as either congenital or acquired. Acquired deformities arise post-traumatically after surgery for lung cancer or a pneumonectomy. Some deformities are associated with spinal malformations, for example kyphosis, it can also be part and parcel of other defects such as Marfan's syndrome. The most common congenital defect is pectus excavatum; this can be severe in some cases and occasionally leads to minimal depression. Symptoms are not always visible in every case. Most severe cases present intolerance to exercise, pain and fatigue. Psychological impact is seen amongst patients due to cosmetic appearance, and this can affect day-to-day working and cause distress socially: finding problems with friendship, relationships and sometimes can affect self-esteem and confidence. Treatment options were invasive initially, using skeletal correction techniques. Now, more minimally invasive procedures are carried out to return the sternum to normal position.

Pectus excavatum is described as a congenital deformity of the anterior chest wall, caused by excessive growth of the connective tissue uniting the sternum and adjacent ribs. The sternal body is depressed and sunken at the xiphisternal junction. The lower costal cartilages buckle inwards to form the depression. Pectus excavatum is relatively common and observed in one in every 400 live births with a male: female ratio of 4:1. In 15–40 % of cases there is a close relative on either side of the family with the same deformity, and a higher preponderance among Caucasians is observed. It is far more frequent than other connective tissue abnormalities. For example, Marfan's syndrome is observed in one in every 5000 live births, and Noonan's syndrome is observed in one in every 2500 live births.

The compression of the sternum limits thoracic volume and therefore vital capacity, negatively impacting exercise tolerance and endurance during cardiovascular exercise. In some cases, cardiac compression is observed. This causes a significant reduction in cardiac output further contributing to exercise intolerance and fatigue. Postoperative research has been undertaken to prove that surgical intervention has significantly benefitted patients' respiratory function and exercise tolerance.

Furthermore, pectus excavatum has profound effects on the psychological state of the individual suffering with the deformity. Pectus excavatum patients suffer frequent embarrassment over physical appearance and teasing by childhood peers. The typical patient starts to become aware of the condition at the onset of puberty, and this has detrimental effects on the individual's confidence and happiness in early adolescence. In fact, 80 % of patients undergoing treatment admitted to suffering with psychological limitations concerning attractiveness, self-esteem and somatisation. In severe cases, some individuals may retreat from society and cease to socialise with peers or participate in exposing sporting activities, such as swimming. This led to the labelling of pectus excavatum as a psychosomatic disorder and further merited surgical and non-surgical intervention.

There are many modes of treatment from braces to implants with varying success. The NUSS procedure which was introduced by Prof. Donald Nuss was initially offered to children, but recently more adult patients have been offered this with exceptional results. In this book we shall discuss the common treatments and options with one of the experts in the field.

Initially, the deformity was surgically corrected through the Ravitch procedure. Now, more commonly, the Nuss procedure is undertaken to readjust and advance the sternal position with the use of a concave steel bar inserted retrosternal through bilateral incisions. The intervention has very few documented side effects but causes marginal postoperative pain that varies amongst individuals. The pain is usually mild and short lasting; however, effective pain management greatly influences a patient's satisfaction and perspective on the success of the treatment. Pain management differs amongst institutions with the majority using thoracic epidurals. Few institutions utilise patient controlled anaesthesia, and these centres believe that it should become the more widely used option postoperatively as it decreases the length of hospitalisation after the intervention. The 'minimally invasive' Nuss procedure is growing in popularity due to infrequent complications, very few side effects and a short length of hospitalisation, lasting 3–4 days, post-operation.

The following chapters will outline various aspects of the management, treatment and consequences of the disorder. Our aim is to provide information around the different treatment options available, their possible complications and future necessities for public education.

Contents

Contributors

Elizabeth M.C. Ashley, BSc, MBChB, FRCA, FFICM Department of Anesthesia and Cardiothoracic Intensive Care, The Heart Hospital UCLH, London, UK

Frank-Martin Haecker, MD, FEAPU Department of Pediatric Surgery, University Children's Hospital, Basel, Switzerland

Dawn E. Jaroszewski, MD, MBA, FACS Department of Cardiothoracic Surgery, Mayo Clinic Arizona, Phoenix, AZ, USA

Kevin J. Johnson, MD Department of General Surgery, Mayo Clinic Arizona, Phoenix, AZ, USA

Shyam K. Kolvekar, MS, MCh, FRCS, FRCSCTh Department of Cardiothoracic Surgery, University College London Hospitals, The Heart Hospital and Barts Heart Center, London, UK

Trupti Kolvekar, BSc Biochemistry (Hon) The Department of Structural Molecular Biology, University College London, London, UK

Marie Maagaard, PhD Student Department of Cardiothoracic and Vascular Surgery, Aarhus University Hospital, Aarhus, Denmark

Department of Clinical Medicine, Aarhus University Hospital, Aarhus, Denmark

Marcelo Martinez-Ferro, MD Department of Surgery, Fundacion Hospitalaria Children's Hospital, Buenos Aires, Argentina

Nikolaos Panagiotopoulos, MD, PhD Department of Cardiothoracic Surgery, University College London Hospitals (UCLH), London, UK

Robert A. Pearl, MD, FRCS(Plast) Department of Plastic and Reconstructive Surgery, Queen Victoria Hospital, East Grinstead, UK

Hans K. Pilegaard, MD Associate Professor, Department of Cardiothoracic and Vascular Surgery, Department of Clinical Medicine, Aarhus University Hospital, Denmark, Aarhus, Denmark

Rajeev Shukla, MChem(Hons), MB, BS(Lon) Department of Cardiothoracic Surgery, The Heart Hospital, University College London Hospital NHS Trust, London, UK

Natalie L. Simon, MBBS Department of School of Medical Education, Kings College London, London, UK

Simon Withey, MBBS, FRCS FRCS(Ed) FRCS(Plast) Department of Plastic and Reconstructive Surgery, The Royal Free Hospital, University College Hospital London, London, UK

Herbert J. Witzke, MD Department of Cardiothoracic Surgery, University Hospital College London, London, UK

Mustafa Yuksel, MD, PhD Department of Thoracic Surgery, Marmara University Hospital, Istanbul, Turkey

Introduction

1

Shyam K. Kolvekar

Abstract

Among all chest wall deformities Pectus Excavatum (PE) or funnel chest represents the most common congenital chest wall deformity accounting for 90 % of all deformities. Pectus Carinatum (PC) or protrusion deformity of the chest wall accounts for 5 % of all chest wall deformities affecting 1 in 2500 live births. Surgical intervention has significantly benefitted patient respiratory function and exercisetolerance. Initially, the deformity was surgically corrected through the Ravitch procedure The introduction of the NUSS procedure in 1998 for the surgical correction of pectus excavatum was the beginning of a new era for the management of chest wall deformities.

Keywords

Pectus Excavatum (PE) • Pectus Carinatum (PC) • Ravitch procedure • NUSS procedure

Pectus excavatum is described as a congenital deformity of the anterior chest wall, caused by excessive growth of the connective tissue uniting the sternum and adjacent ribs. The sternal body is depressed and sunken at the xiphisternal junction. The lower costal cartilages buckle inwards to form the depression. Pectus excavatum is relatively common and observed in one in every 400 live births with a male: female ratio of 4:1. In 15–40 % of cases there is a close relative on either side of the family with the same deformity and a higher preponderance among Caucasians is observed. It is far more frequent than other connective tissue abnormalities. For example, Marfan's syndrome is observed in one in every 5,000 live births and Noonan's syndrome is observed in one in every 2,500 live births (Fig. 1.1). Pectus excavatum is categorised as an idiopathic abnormality, however research has been conducted to hypothesise genetic defect. Other postulated hypotheses exist for the pathogenesis of PE; developmental disorders or

S.K. Kolvekar, MS, MCh, FRCS, FRCSCTh
Department of Cardiothoracic Surgery,
University College London Hospitals, The Heart
Hospital and Barts Heart Center, London, UK
e-mail: kolvekar@yahoo.com

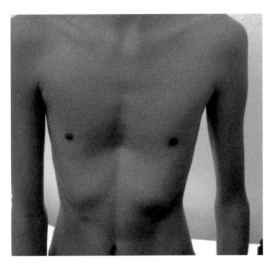

Fig. 1.1 Pectus excavatum

cartilage overgrowth. Although both may contribute to the deformation, in further chapters we present another hypothesis relating to genetic in growth factor-like signaling molecule involved in the uniting of sternal cartilage and adjacent ribs.

The compression of the sternum limits thoracic volume and therefore vital capacity, negatively impacting exercise tolerance and endurance during cardiovascular exercise. In some cases, cardiac compression is observed. This causes a significant reduction in cardiac output further contributing to exercise intolerance and fatigue.

Surgical intervention has significantly benefitted patient respiratory function and exercise tolerance. Initially, the deformity was surgically corrected through the Ravitch procedure. Now, more commonly, the Nuss procedure is undertaken to readjust and advance the sternal position with the use of a concave steel bar inserted retrosternal through bilateral incisions. The intervention has very few documented side effects but causes marginal postoperative pain that varies amongst individuals. The pain is usually mild and short-lasting, however, effective pain management greatly influences a patient's satisfaction and perspective on the success of the treatment. Pain management differs amongst institutions with the majority using thoracic epidurals. Few institutions utilise patient controlled anaesthesia and these centres believe that it

should become the more widely used option postoperatively as it decreases the length of hospitalisation after the intervention (Fig. 1.2).

The introduction of the NUSS procedure in 1998 for the surgical correction of pectus excavatum was the beginning of a new era for the management of chest wall deformities and a new significant chapter in the modern Thoracic Surgery [1]. The 'minimally-invasive' Nuss procedure is growing in popularity due to infrequent complications, very few side effects and a short length of hospitalisation, lasting 2–4 days, post-operation (Fig. 1.3).

Furthermore, pectus excavatum has profound effects on the psychological state of the individual suffering with the deformity. Pectus excavatum patients suffer frequent embarrassment over physical appearance and teasing by childhood peers. The typical patient starts to become aware of the condition at the onset of puberty and this has detrimental effects on the individual's confidence and happiness in early adolescence. In fact, 80 % of patients undergoing treatment admitted to suffering with psychological limitations concerning attractiveness, self-esteem and somatization. In severe cases, some individuals may retreat from society and cease to socialize with peers or participate in exposing sporting activities, such as swimming. This led to the labeling of pectus excavatum as a psychosomatic disorder and further merited surgical and non-surgical intervention.

Over the decades different studies revealed that most of deformities are familiar with a strong genetic involvement and usually related with other syndromes, anomalies and defects making the management challenging [2]. Nevertheless the majority of chest wall anomalies remain rare clinical entities and some of them like thoracic ectopia cordis are not compatible with life and very unlikely to be benefited by a surgical procedure [3]. The approach of chest wall deformities is still controversial as it's not the clinical symptoms – mainly cardiopulmonary – but also the psychosocial aspects and effects of poor cosmetic that have a huge impact to the quality of life [4]. For that reason in recent years has been a significant increase in the interest of clinicians for assessment and management of these patients.

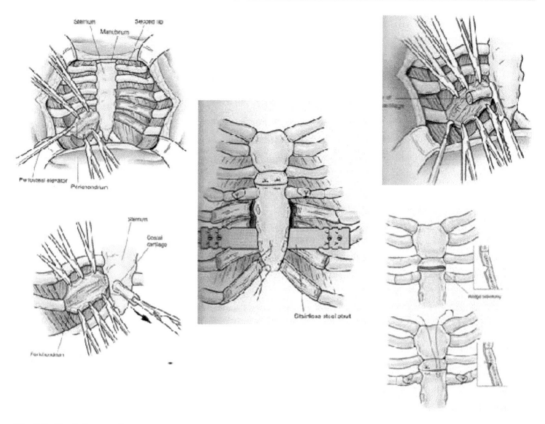

Fig. 1.2 Ravitch procedure

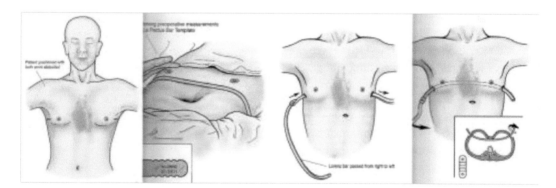

Fig. 1.3 NUSS procedure

Toward that direction new assessment criteria have been established and new minimally invasive surgical techniques have been introduced. Different classifications have been proposed through years to categories chest wall anomalies. In 2006 Acastello classified them into five types depending on the site of origin of the anomaly (type I: cartilagineous, type II: costal, type III: chondro-costal, type IV: sternal, type V: clavicle-scapular) [5].

Among all chest wall deformities Pectus Excavatum (PE) or funnel chest represents the most common congenital chest wall deformity accounting for 90 % of all deformities [6]. The first description came from Bauhinus1 in the sixteenth century [7] and main characteristic is the depression of sternum and lower cartilages [8] with an incidence between 1 and 8 per 1000 children [9].

Pectus Carinatum (PC) or protrusion deformity of the chest wall accounts for 5 % of all chest wall deformities affecting 1 in 2500 live births [10]. It can be unilateral, bilateral or mixed and there is predominance in males (Fig. 1.4) [11].

Pectus arcuatum represents a rare category of chest wall deformities in the family of pectus anomalies and It includes mixed excavatum and carinatum features along a longitudinal or transversal axis resulting in a multiplanar curvature of the sternum and adjacent ribs (Fig. 1.5) [12].

Poland syndrome (PS) is classified as a chondrocostal chest wall deformity with main clinical manifestation the underdevelopment or absence of the major pectorals muscle [13]. Is a congenital unilateral chest wall deformity that affects both males and females in a ratio of 3:1 and with an incident variation from 1 to 70,000 to 1 to 100,000 live births [14].

Sternal cleft represents a rare idiopathic chest wall deformity caused by a defect in the sternum's fusion process. It accounts for 0.15 % of all chest wall deformities [15] and there is an a association with the Hexb gene [16]. There are four types of sternal clefts according to the classification proposed by Schamberger and Welch in 1990 [17].

Jeune Syndrome, also known as Asphyxiating Thoracic Dystrophy (ATD) is a rare autosomal recessive skeletal dysplasia with multiorgan involvement. It was first described by Jeune et al. [18] in 1954 and it affects 1 per 10,0000 to 13,0000 live births [19]. There are two subtypes of the syndrome with severe subtype being incompatible with life [20].

The following chapters will outline various aspects of the management, treatment and consequences of the disorder. Our aim is to provide information around the different treatment options available, their possible complications and future necessities for public education.

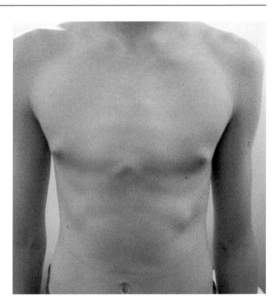

Fig. 1.4 Pectus carinatum

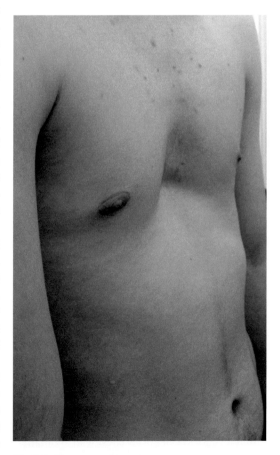

Fig. 1.5 Pectus arcuatum

References

1. Nuss D, Kelly Jr RE, Croitoru DP, Katz ME. A 10-year review of a minimally invasive technique for the correction of pectus excavatum. J Pediatr Surg. 1998;33(4):545–52.
2. Kelly Jr RE, Shamberger RC, Mellins RB, Mitchell KK, Lawson ML, Oldham K, et al. Prospective multicenter study of surgical correction of pectus excavatum: design, perioperative complications, pain, and baseline pulmonary function facilitated by internet-based data collection. J Am Coll Surg. 2007;205:205–16.
3. Dobell AR, Williams HB, Long RW. Staged repair of ectopia cordis. J Pediatr Surg. 1982;17(4):353–8.
4. Colombani PM. Preoperative assessment of chest wall deformities. Semin Thorac Cardiovasc Surg. 2009;21:58–63.
5. Acastello E. Patologias de la pared toracica en pediatria. Buenos Aires: Editorial El Ateneo; 2006.
6. Kotzot D, Schwabegger AH. Etiology of chest wall deformities—a genetic review for the treating physician. J Pediatr Surg. 2009;44:2004–11.
7. Bauhinus J. Johannes Observatorium medicarum, rararum, novarum, admirabilium, et montrosarum, liber secundus. In: Ioannis Schenckii a Grafenberg, editor. Observation. Frankfurt: De partibus vitalibus, thorace contentis; 1609. p. 322.
8. Fonkalsrud EW, Dunn JC, Atkinson JB. Repair of pectus excavatum deformities: 30 years of experience with 375 patients. Ann Surg. 2000;231:443–8.
9. Kelly Jr RE, Lawson ML, Paidas CN, Hruban RH. Pectus excavatum in a 112-year autopsy series: anatomic findings and the effect on survival. J Pediatr Surg. 2005;40:1275–8.
10. Nuss D, Croitoru DP, Kelly RE. Congenital chest wall deformities. In: Ashcraft KW, Holcomb III GW, Murphy JP, editors. Pediatric Surgery. 4th ed. Philadelphia: Elsevier Saunders; 2005. p. 245–63.
11. Shamberger RC, Welch KJ. Surgical correction of pectus carinatum. J Pediatr Surg. 1987;22:48–53.
12. Duhamel P, Brunel C, Le Pimpec F, Pons F, Jancovici R. Correction of the congenital malformations of the front chest by the modelling technique of sternochondroplasty: technique and results on a series of 14 cases. Ann Chir Plast Esthet. 2003;48:77–85.
13. Clarkson P. Poland's syndactyly. Guys Hosp Rep. 1962;111:335–46.
14. Fokin A, Robicsek F. Poland's syndrome revisited. Ann Thorac Surg. 2002;74(6):2218.
15. Acastello E, Majluf F, Garrido P, Barbosa LM, Peredo A. Sternal cleft: a surgical opportunity. J Pediatr Surg. 2003;38(2):178–83.
16. Forzano F, Daubeney PE, White SM. (2005) Midline raphe, sternal cleft, and other midline abnormalities: a new dominant syndrome? Am J Med Genet A. 2005;135(1):9–12.
17. Shamberger R, Welch K. Sternal defects. Pediatr Surg Int. 1990;5:156–64.
18. Jeune M, Carron R, Beraud C, Loaec Y. Polychondrodystrophie avec blocage thoracique d'évolution fatale. Pediatrie. 1954;9(4):390–2.
19. Oberklaid F, Danks DM, Mayne V, Campbell P. Asphyxiating thoracic dysplasia. Clinical, radiological, and pathological information on 10 patients. Arch Dis Child. 1977;52(10):758–65.
20. O'Connor MB, Gallagher DP, Mulloy E. Jeune syndrome. Postgrad Med J. 2008;84:559.

Shyam K. Kolvekar, Natalie L. Simon,
and Trupti Kolvekar

Abstract

In Pectus Excavatum, the sternum is cast-down and depressed into a convex shape. The sternal malformation is caused by the extensive growth of the costal cartilages, inserting into the sternal body. The growth allows the cartilages to clump together and further push the sternum inwards. Having an appendicular derivative, the sternum develops from two sternal bar components. The following chapter aims to evaluate the embryological contributing factors to the development of Pectus Excavatum.

Keywords

Chest wall deformity • Pectus Excavatum • Sternum • Malformation • Costal cartilages • Epidemiology

Developmental Anatomy of Pectus Excavatum

In pectus excavatum, the sternum is cast-down and depressed into a convex shape. The sternal malformation is caused by the extensive growth of the costal cartilages, inserting into the sternal body.

S.K. Kolvekar, MS, MCh, FRCS, FRCSCTh (✉)
Department of Cardiothoracic Surgery,
University College London Hospitals, The Heart
Hospital and Barts Heart Center, London, UK
e-mail: kolvekar@yahoo.com

N.L. Simon, MBBS
Department of School of Medical Education,
Kings College London, London, UK

T. Kolvekar, BSc Biochemistry (Hon)
The Department of Structural Molecular Biology,
University College London, London, UK

The growth allows the cartilages to clump together and further push the sternum inwards. Many pathophysiological hypotheses exist regarding the primary cause of pectus excavatum. These hypotheses refer to intrauterine mechanical factors, respiratory muscular imbalance in diseases like Spinal Muscular Atrophy type I and developmental delays being responsible. Present day theories centralise on the cause being a developmental disorder, allied with maturation disturbances of the sternocostal cartilage. To further support this hypothesis, histological changes in the sternocostal cartilage of those with pectus excavatum were observed [1]. Another instance of rib malformation is the cervical rib. This occurs when the thoracic wall of adults is arranged in an oblique manner, with the ribs angled forwards and downwards in an unorthodox fashion.

© Springer International Publishing Switzerland 2016
S.K. Kolvekar, H.K. Pilegaard (eds.), *Chest Wall Deformities and Corrective Procedures*,
DOI 10.1007/978-3-319-23968-2_2

Embryological Development of the Thoracic Cage and Sternal Development

Having an appendicular derivative, the sternum develops from two sternal bar components. The sternum develops independently of both ribs and the pectoral girdle. It originates in the lateral somatopleuric mesoderm, from the ventro-medial sclerotome at the body wall and forms as a pair of mesenchymal condensations. The pair of cranio-caudally orientated sternal bars assemble alongside the midline and fuse to form the cartilaginous model of the manubrium, sternabrae and xiphoid process (the three main components of the sternum). The primary ossification centres of the all parts of the sternum, excluding the xiphoid process, appear before

birth. With respect to the xiphoid process, the centre of ossification is observed during childhood. In the case of incomplete fusion of the respective parts of the sternum, perforation becomes a major issue. Development of the sternal body begins in the 6th gestational week. The sternal primordia (tissue in early development) move towards each other and protract to congregate into sternal bars that make contact with the primordial ribs. The sternal bars commence fusing at the manubrium's midline and proceed chondrify to a cartilaginous model by week 10 (Fig. 2.1) [2].

The caudal extension of the sternal bars forms the xiphoid process. The segmentation of the mesosternum into the sternal body is influenced by the ribs and their respective attachment sites [3].

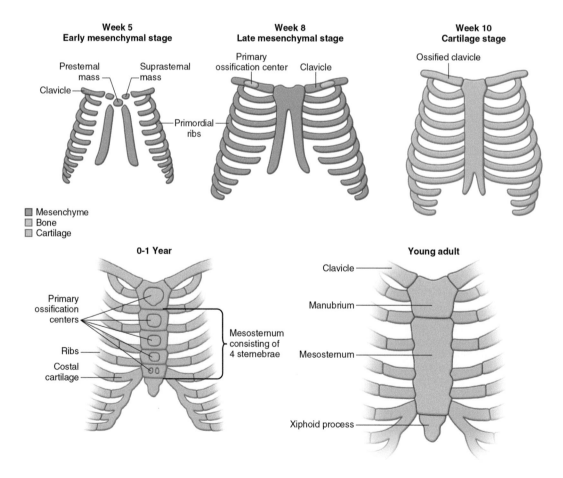

Fig. 2.1 Embryologic and postnatal development of the human sternum [2]

There are cases where the centre of ossification evolves before sternal bar component fusion. These centres of ossification can form in both bars. Conventionally, ossification of the sternum is much later than fusion; it begins during the 5th gestational month. The manubrium is the first to ossify, whereas the last to ossify is the xiphoid process. This stage of development only begins after 3 years of age – the age can be variable [4].

Rib Development

The ribs are also derived from the sclerotome portion of the paraxial mesoderm that forms the vertebrae's costal processes. They form as elongations of the costal process of the thoracic vertebrae. Primary ossification centers appear in the body of the ribs at 14 weeks of development. The ribs are more horizontal in the infant, with less curvature, in comparison to the adult. The secondary ossification centres appear at the rib's tubercle during puberty. Ribs 1–7 (referred to as true ribs) attach to the sternum through their own cartilages. The false ribs [5–8] attach to the sternum by the cartilage of another rib or adjacent ribs and the floating ribs don't attach to the sternum [1, 9]. The costal cartilages' embryological origin is through migrating sclerotome cells that move from the lateral somatic boundary into the lateral plate mesoderm. The costal cartilages join the sternal end of the ribs and then attach to the sternum at articular facets. Sternocostal joints formed here are synovial and are supported by ligaments that anchor the costal cartilages to the sternal sides. Articular cavities are commonly replaced by fibrocartilage, however, and are known as chondrosternal joints. The ribs attach when the fusion of sternum bars are complete; the sternal tissue band guides the formation of the ventral part of the rib. It is known that chondroblasts are involved in the development of the sternocostal articulation. Cells from the perichondrium proliferate between the sternum and ribs to form the sternocostal joints [5]. New hypotheses state that a faulty mechanism behind sternocostal joint development is a caus-ative factor for congenital chest wall deformities and sternal depressions.

Similarities and Differences in Thoracic Development in Humans, Compared to Other Animals

Moreover, the vertebral column is derived from the somatic sclerotomes, whereas the ribs are formed by condensations of sclerotomal cells and the intercostal muscles are derived from the dermomyotomes [6]. Additionally, the distal parts of the ribs have been found to partially originate from the dermomyotomes [7]. Kato and Aoyama concluded that these findings were linked to the removal and the transplantation of the dermomyotomes in avian embryos. The results of R. Huang et al. disagree and show, with clarity, the proximal and the distal parts of the ribs being formed by the sclerotomal mesenchyme. Huang et al. go on to explain that Kato and Aoyama's interpretation was due to a grafting technique in which three consecutive thoracic dermomyotomes with adjacent lateral plate mesoderm were grafted together. R. Huang's method avoided the inclusion of sclerotomal cells into the graft by isolating a single dermomyotomes. The study also concludes that morphogenic Pax-1 protein is required for the formation of the proximal ribs. This is reinforced in a study by Braun et al., stating that the distal parts are missing in Myf5 and Pax-3 deficient mice. In a contrasting study by Wallin et al., the proximal ribs are not apparent in Pax-1 deleted mice [6]. Formation of the distal ribs may, therefore, depend on communication between the sclerotome and myotome. Both studies were conducted on mice, which have a similar embryological development to humans.

The formation of vertebrae and ribs in veterinary medicine is alike that in human medicine. Somite sclerotomes migrate to surround the neural tube as a mass. This mass proceeds to create a cartilaginous model. The diffuse region of one somite joins with the dense region of another neighbouring somite. Sclerotome mesenchyme forms annulus fibrous (outer coating of the intervertebral disc) and the notochord forms the nucleus pulposus (gel substance filling the spinal disc). The ribs then are developments from the thoracic vertebral processes.

Mammals have thoracic vertebral ribs only. Marsupials and placental mammals, on the other hand, have cervical and lumbar ribs that are found only as remnants fused to vertebral transverse processes. Birds have most of their ribs in the thoracic region with the exception of small fused cervical ribs. Fish have two sets of ribs attached to the vertebral column. The dorsal ribs are found in the septal area in between inferior and superior musculature and project sideways. In contrast, the ventral ribs begin caudal to the dorsal ribs. Sharks only have short ventral ribs and lack a dorsal set. Between amphibians and reptiles, there is variation in rib number. Turtles have eight pairs of ribs. These ribs form a plastron, which constitutes the flat part of a turtle's shell and a cartilaginous carapace in the upper exoskeleton. Frogs have no ribs, except for a functional sacral pair forming the pelvis and allowing for stabilisation of movement. Surprisingly, dogs have 26 ribs. A Pekingese dog with hemivertebrae, rib malformations and spinal cord dysraphism (without spina bifida) was documented in a mid-90s study. Thoracic hemivertebrae was observed alongside anomalies of the dorsal median septum. To conclude, the dog showed malformations of the vertebral regions and ribs from mesodermal origin. Spinal dysraphism is of ectodermic origin, when considering embryological defaults. This suggests that mammalian thoracic defaults, between humans and dogs, can possibly be explained by embryological developmental problems [8].

Epidemiology

The prevalence of Pectus excavatum is estimated to be between 0.1 and 0.8 % of the cohort examined [5]. A large autopsy series conducted to esti-mate the incidence of pectus excavatum and other associated conditions has concluded a value lower than Brochhausen et al. of 0.12 %. Following survival analysis, it was found that pectus excavatum patients had a noticeable tendency to die earlier than the control group evaluated (P=.0001). In contrast, it was also found that the pectus excavatum patients who survived past the age of 56 years, survived longer than the same control group (P=.0001) [9]. A frequent birth prevalence estimate is 0.25 % (1/400 people) and pectus carinatum is two to four times less common than pectus excavatum [1]. A male to female predominance of pectus excavatum exists at a ratio of 5:1 or higher. In 15–40 % of cases there is a close relative on either side of the family with the same deformity. A higher preponderance among Caucasians was also found; out of all patients with idiopathic pectus excavatum studied in a teaching hospital in the USA, 89 % were Caucasians, 9 % were Hispanic and only 2 % were Asian [10]. The chest deformity is rare in Africa and authors have only observed 10 African-American patients out of more than 1000 patients studied. Furthermore, pectus excavatum comprises 87 % of chest wall deformities. Although this is the majority, pectus excavatum is linked with a number of associated ailments. For example, it is estimated that 19 % of pectus excavatum patients had clinical features suggestive of Marfan's syndrome. Males have an increased risk of this deformity and females have an increased risk of associated scoliosis (scoliosis was identified in 29 % of patients.) In addition, Ehlers-Danlos syndrome was present in another 2.1 % of patients [11]. Eighty-six percent of PE cases are discerned in the first year of life and the majority of the remaining cases present in early adolescence. It is uncommon for resolution of the depression to occur spontaneously during this period and the depression is found to worsen during puberty [12]. There are limited family studies conducted to evaluate and determine the inheritance pattern of pectus excavatum. Creswick et al., however, surveyed 34 families and the majority (41 %) were found to display autosomal dominant inheritance. Autosomal recessive inheritance was apparent in 12 % and X-chromosomal inheritance in 18 % of families [13].

Probable Causes of Chest Wall Deformity

Causation of chest wall deformities is multifactorial. The condition is commonly associated with several genetic syndromes. Bauhinus first suggested an increase in diaphragmatic pressure, seen during embryonic development, to be a principal pathophysiologic attributing factor [5]. One opinion was that intrauterine pressure on the sternum through an abnormal position of the embryo could lead to repositioning and subsequent deformation [14]. Following viewpoints called upon permanent mechanical stress through extreme repositioning to be the main causative factor.

Brown published observations of sternal retraction due to a thickening of the ligamentum substernale [15–18]. Some suggested an imbalance between the anterior and posterior formation of muscle fibres of the anterior part of the diaphragm to cause sternal regression and further xiphoid movement. Other hypotheses discuss diseases such as syphilis or rickets as contributing factors to pectus excavatum (PE).

Studies assessing the histological changes in sternocostal cartilage in PE patients reveal premature ageing of the cartilage. Biochemical studies demonstrate decreased levels of zinc and increased levels of magnesium and calcium in the costal cartilages of PE patients. Reasons given for this observation are that zinc deficiency results in lower chondrocyte metabolic activity. Feng et al.'s study concluded a correlation between metabolic lesions and mechanical strength of the cartilage [18].

Most recent focus is on biomechanical weakness caused by an insufficient sternocostal cartilage metabolism. Nakaoka et al. showed that the costal cartilage on the side of deepest impression has no correlation with that of the contralateral side [16]. On the contrary, Fokin et al., found matrix disorganization in the cartilage of PE patients and suggested that to be the reason for sternal cartilage overgrowth [17].

In conclusion, both cartilaginous overgrowth and developmental disorders may contribute to the development of PE and other chest wall deformities.

My Hypothesis

I would like to propose the following hypothesis, stating that a growth factor-like signaling molecule is responsible for the rate and extent to which sternal cartilage and ribs unite. If there is a defect in the signaling pathway due to a mutation in one of the growth receptors or paracrine signals, the cartilage is either pushed forward or compressed downwards, leading to malformation and re-positioning (Fig. 2.2).

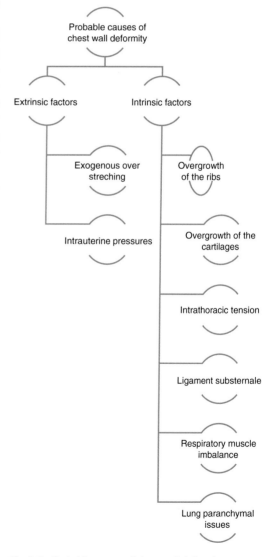

Fig. 2.2 Probable causes of chest wall deformity

References

1. Cobben JM, Oostra RJ, van Dijk FS. Pectus excavatum and carinatum. Eur J Med Genet. 2014;57(8):414–7.
2. van der Merwe AE, Weston DA, Oostra RJ, Maat GJ. A review of the embryological development and associated developmental abnormalities of the sternum in the light of a rare palaeopathological case of sternal clefting. Homo. 2013;64(2):129–41.
3. Barnes E. Developmental defects of the axial skeleton in paleopathology. Niwat: University Press of Colorado; 1994.
4. Scheuer L, Black S. The juvenile skeleton. Amsterdam: Elsevier/Academic; 2004.
5. Brochhausen C, Turial S, Müller FK, et al. Pectus excavatum: history, hypotheses and treatment options. Interact Cardiovasc Thorac Surg. 2012;14(6): 801–6.
6. Huang R, Zhi Q, Schmidt C, Wilting J, Brand-Saberi B, Christ B. Sclerotomal origin of the ribs. Development. 2000;127(3):527–32.
7. Kato N, Aoyama H. Dermomyotomal origin of the ribs as revealed by extirpation and transplantation experiments in chick and quail embryos. Development. 1998;125(17):3437–43.
8. Ruberte J, Añor S, Carretero A, et al. Malformations of the vertebral bodies and the ribs associated to spinal dysraphism without spina bifida in a Pekingese dog. Zentralbl Veterinarmed A. 1995;42(5):307–13.
9. Kelly Jr RE, Lawson ML, Paidas CN, Hruban RH. Pectus excavatum in a 112-year autopsy series: anatomic findings and the effect on survival. J Pediatr Surg. 2005;40(8):1275–8.
10. Koumbourlis AC. Pectus excavatum: pathophysiology and clinical characteristics. Paediatr Respir Rev. 2009;10(1):3–6.
11. Kelly Jr RE, Croitoru D, Nuss D. Chest wall anomalies: pectus excavatum and pectus carinatum. Adolesc Med Clin. 2004;15(3):455–71.
12. Obermeyer RJ, Goretsky MJ. Chest wall deformities in pediatric surgery. Surg Clinic North Am. 2012;92(3):669–84.
13. Kotzot D, Schwabegger AH. Etiology of chest wall deformities—a genetic review for the treating physician. J Pediatr Surg. 2009;44(10):2004–11.
14. Williams CT. Congenital malformation of the thorax great depression of the sternum. Trans Path Soc. 1872;24:50.
15. Brown AL. Pectus excavatum (funnel chest). J Thorac Surg. 1939;9:164–84.
16. Nakaoka T, Uemura S, Yano T, Nakagawa Y, Tanimoto T, Suehiro S. Does overgrowth of costal cartilage cause pectus excavatum? A study on the lengths of ribs and costal cartilages in asymmetric patients. J Pediatr Surg. 2009;44:1333–6.
17. Fokin AA, Robicsek F, Watts LT. Genetic analysis of connective tissue in patients with congenital thoracic abnormalities. Interact Cardiovasc Thorac Surg. 2008;7:56.
18. Feng J, Hu T, Liu W, Zhang S, Tang Y, Chen R, et al. The biomechanical, morphologic, and histochemical properties of the costal cartilages in children with pectus excavatum. J Pediatr Surg. 2001;36:1770–6.

History

Natalie L. Simon, Trupti Kolvekar, and
Shyam K. Kolvekar

Abstract

Bauhinus produced the cardinal definition of a funnel-form chest in the sixteenth century. He assessed the clinical features of pectus excavatum in a patient suffering with pulmonary compression, dyspnea (shortness of breath) and paroxysmal cough; the symptoms appraised by Bauhinus aided the embellishment of his definition of the deformation. The Nuss procedure to correct the deformity relies on two interventions: the first, to insert the steel bar through bilateral anterior-axillary thoracic incisions and the second, to remove the bar after 3 years.

Keywords

Chest wall deformity • Pectus Excavatum • Funnel-form chest • Nuss Procedure • Ravitch Procedure

Bauhinus produced the cardinal definition of a funnel-form chest in the sixteenth century. He assessed the clinical features of pectus excavatum in a patient suffering with pulmonary compression, dyspnea (shortness of breath) and paroxysmal cough; the symptoms appraised by Bauhinus aided the embellishment of his definition of the deformation [1]. Another documented observation of thoracic abnormality followed in the mid-1800s by Woillez. The work of von Luschka and Eggel then followed, instigating the publication of the first ever comprehensive case report of a funnel-formed thorax depression; the case report was named 'miraculum naturae.' Eggel and other scholars at the time relied on the assumption that the condition is engendered by sternal inflexibility due to malnutrition or developmental defects. Hagmann superseded with an alternative hypothesis, stating the cause of pectus excavatum to be closely linked with the overgrowth of the ribs. In fact,

N.L. Simon, MBBS
Department of School of Medical Education,
Kings College London, London, UK

T. Kolvekar, BSc Biochemistry (Hon)
The Department of Structural Molecular Biology,
University College London, London, UK

S.K. Kolvekar, MS, MCh, FRCS, FRCSCTh (✉)
The Department of Structural Molecular Biology,
University College London Hospitals, The Heart Hospital and Barts Heart Center, London, UK
e-mail: kolvekar@yahoo.com

© Springer International Publishing Switzerland 2016
S.K. Kolvekar, H.K. Pilegaard (eds.), *Chest Wall Deformities and Corrective Procedures*,
DOI 10.1007/978-3-319-23968-2_3

surgical interventionists believed that rib cartilage removal would be successful in correcting the abnormal sternum positioning [2]. Further case reports (one documenting five patients) materialised in nineteenth century by Ebstein. During this time period, patients were prescribed *"Fresh air, breathing exercises, aerobic activities and lateral pressure"* in order to improve respiratory function. Present day clinical practice calls on early correctional interventions by advising patients to partake in various rehabilitation exercises, subsequently benefitting posture. In addition, the figure-of-eight clavicular fracture splint is still utilised as a correctional technique. The First World War saw substantial advances in endotracheal intubation, improving ventilator prospects. Prior to this, only limited corrections could be carried out [3]. Genetics as a predisposing factor for pectus excavatum was discovered by Coulson in 1820; his study investigated three siblings with the deformity [4]. Recently studying one of Leonardo da Vinci's images from 1510, Ashraflan note for the first time that there is an image of pectus excavatum (Fig. 3.1) in an elderly individual [5].

The first operation to correct pectus excavatum was conducted in 1911 by Meyer. The intention of

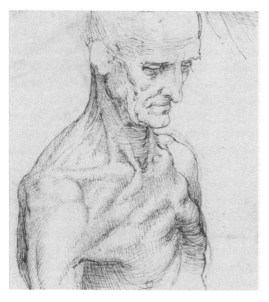

Fig. 3.1 Image of the upper thorax demonstrating pectus excavatum. Leonardo da Vinci, circa 1510–1511 (Supplied by Royal Collection Trust/© HM Queen Elizabeth II 2013)

the surgical intercession was to remove rib cartilage. This reinforced the earlier hypothesis of rib overgrowth, being the ascendant predisposing factor, laid out by Hagmann. Meyer removed the second to third costal cartilages on the right side of the chest wall. There was no significant improvement and the operation was deemed unsuccessful [2]. Sauerbruch pioneered twentieth century treatments by incising and excoriating the left 5th to 9th costal cartilages and a section of the adjacent sternum. The surgery was proven to alleviate symptoms of dyspnea and allowed the patient to return to normal life relatively quickly [6]. A few years later, Sauerbruch begun the first consummate pectus correction through subperichondrial resection of all deformed cartilage and sternal stabilization using bar implantation. This operation required excessively invasive retrosternal dissection and transversal osteotomies [2]. Ravitch elucidated and presented the following steps for the surgical correction of pectus excavatum. He described the initial step of a bilateral parasternal and subperichondrial resection of affected costal cartilages, followed by the detachment of the xiphoid process. Further, he outlined the use of transverse wedge osteotomy at the upper edge of the sternal depression and the re-placement of the sternum anteriorly- in order to secure its place. Numerous methods of repair followed Ravitch's outlines [7].

Sauerbruch's technique was universalized by Ravitch and preceded revolutionary interventions uncovered by Nuss in 1998. Nuss' technique was contrastive to others developed earlier in the fact that it was minimally invasive. The procedure operates through the insertion of a steel bar through bilateral anterior-axillary thoracic incisions under thoracoscopic guidance- to highlight the pathway taken by the metal bar [8]. The bar advances to the contralateral side prior to it being pulled through the anterior incisions. At the second procedure (after 2 years), the lateral incisions made to insert the bar are entered and the stabilisers attached to the bar are removed [9]. The steel bar is inserted with convexity facing posteriorly and it is flipped over when in correct positioning. The bar is usually kept in for 2 years to allow for permanent correction and cartilaginous remodeling [10]. The bar is attached to the lateral muscles of the chest wall and is positioned through the use of a stabiliser on either the right side or both sides. In addition, the bar is future cemented to the ribs with subperiosteally-placed cable wires [2]. Other surgical strategies place an external brace, instead of bar, behind the sternum; the Leonard modification is an example of this. This approach incorporates the resection of up to five cartilages and a wedge osteotomy is effectuated, where a wire is positioned behind the sternum and attached to an external brace. Prior to this, the operation requires a curvilinear incision to be made on top of the sternum. To expose the thorax, skin flaps and pectoral muscle flaps are elevated and periosteal elevators are used to dissect the periochondrium from the cartilage. The brace remains in situ for 3 months before removal [9].

Although complications for the Nuss procedure are rare, cardiac perforations from direct cardiac injury have been documented. In addition, pericardial tears are reported in 4.2 % of cases and pericardial effusion in 0.5–2.4 % of cases. Techniques implemented into conventional operations to reduce the risk of cardiac injuries include thoracoscopic guidance and viewing of the mediastinum. Better visualisation of the tip of the dissector or the bar during its passageway through the bilateral incisions and mediastinum has been proven to decrease the rate of direct cardiac injury [11]. Kabbag R et al. carried out a retrospective review of 70 children undergoing the Nuss procedure for correction of pectus excavatum. The data recorded minor complications in 65 % of patients and major complications in 8.5 % of patients. However, no patients experienced major cardiopulmonary or fatal complications. The study concludes the major limitations to thoracoscopic-assisted PE repair to be history of cardio-thoracic surgery and SVD (sternum-to-vertebra distance) sternum rotation angle lower than 5 cm or an SRA greater than 35°, identified through a CT scan. The SVD was measured as the distance from the posterior aspect of the sternum to the anterior aspect of the vertebral body (at the site of greatest deformity depth); the SRA is the angle formed by the horizontal plane and the transverse axis of the sternum, also at the site of greatest deformity depth [12].

The Nuss procedure relies on two interventions: the first, to insert the steel bar through bilateral anterior-axillary thoracic incisions and the second, to remove the bar after 2 years. Future prospects in the field of correctional intervention involve the use of a different bar material. Metal devices were found to migrate into neighbouring tissue and therefore increase postoperative chronic pain. The Strasbourg Thorax Osteosynthesis System (STRATOS®) uses titanium implants to reduce the shift into tissues [2]. STRATOS forms part of numerous novel strategies that erase the requirement for a second intervention. Long-term absorbable stabilisers have recently become available. They are made of poly-L-lactic and polyglycolic acid and aim to reduce postoperative pain and discomfort, by making the removal of the bar easier [13]. Gurkok et al. presented a new technique. Following osteotomy, the sternum is repositioned and a copolymer plaque is placed on top of the sternum. The fixation of the plaque is achieved with reabsorbable polymer screws and a chest tube is inserted if the parietal pleura have been opened. Additionally, a hemovac drain is inserted across the sternum. Gurkok's approach requires a single intervention as none of the factors used in sternal stabilisation are non-absorbable. Studies on the technique report excellent sternal stability. No severe complications in any of the patients studied, after 1-year follow-up, were observed [14].

Epidemiology

The prevalence of Pectus excavatum is estimated to be between 0.1 and 0.8 % of the cohort examined [5]. A large autopsy series conducted to estimate the incidence of pectus excavatum and other associated conditions has concluded a value lower than Brochhausen et al. of 0.12 %. Following survival analysis, it was found that pectus excavatum patients had a noticeable tendency to die earlier than the control group evaluated (P = .0001). In contrast, it was also found that the pectus excavatum patients who survived past the age of 56 years, survived longer than the same control group (P = .0001) [15]. A frequent birth prevalence estimate is 0.25 % (1/400 people) and pectus carinatum is 2–4 times less common than pectus excavatum [16]. A male to female predominance of pectus excavatum exists at a ratio of 5:1 or higher. In 15–40 % of cases there is a close relative on either side of the family with the same deformity. A higher preponderance among Caucasians was also found; out of all patients with idiopathic pectus excavatum studied in a teaching hospital in the USA, 89 % were Caucasians, 9 % were Hispanic and only 2 % were Asian [17]. The chest deformity is rare in Africa and authors have only observed 10 African-American patients out of more than 1000 patients studied. Furthermore, pectus excavatum comprises 87 % of chest wall deformities. Although this is the majority, pectus excavatum is linked with a number of associated ailments. For example, it is estimated that 19 % of pectus excavatum patients had clinical features suggestive of Marfan's syndrome. Males have an increased risk of this deformity and females have an increased risk of associated scoliosis (scoliosis was identified in 29 % of patients). In addition, Ehlers-Danlos syndrome was present in another 2.1 % of patients [18]. Eighty six percent of PE cases are discerned in the first year of life and the majority of the remaining cases present in early adolescence. It is uncommon for resolution of the depression to occur spontaneously during this period and the depression is found to worsen during puberty [19]. There are limited family studies conducted to evaluate and determine the inheritance pattern of pectus excavatum. Creswick et al., however, surveyed 34 families and the majority (41 %) were found to display autosomal dominant inheritance. Autosomal recessive inheritance was apparent in 12 % and X-chromosomal inheritance in 18 % of families [5].

References

1. Bauhinus J. Observationum medicariam. Liber II, observ. 264, Francfurti 1600; p. 507.
2. Brochhausen C, et al. Pectus excavatum: history, hypotheses and treatment options. Interact Cardiovasc Thorac Surg. 2012;14(6):801–6.
3. Kelly RE. Pectus excavatum: historical background, clinical picture, preoperative evaluation and criteria for operation. Semin Pediatr Surg. 2008;17(3):181–93.
4. Coulson W. Deformities of the chest. Lond Med Gaz. 1820;4:69–73.
5. Ashraflan H. Images in thorax. Thorax. 2013;68:1081.
6. Sauerbruch F. Die Chirurgie der Brustorgane. Berlin: Springer; 1920. p. 437.
7. Robicsek F, Watts LT, Fokin AA. Surgical repair of pectus excavatum and carinatum. Semin Thorac Cardiovasc Surg. 2009;21(1):64–75.
8. Huckaby L, Rajeev Prasad R. Minimally invasive repair of pectus excavatum in an adolescent with a history of a median sternotomy as an infant. Journal of Pediatric Surgery Case Reports. 2014;2(10):443–5.
9. Antonoff MB, et al. When patients choose: comparison of Nuss, Ravitch, and Leonard procedures for primary repair of pectus excavatum. J Pediatr Surg. 2009;44(6):1113–9.
10. Nuss D, Kelly RE, Croitoru DP, Katz ME. A 10-year review of a minimally invasive technique for the correction of pectus excavatum. J Pediatr Surg. 1998;33:545–52.
11. Casamassima MGS, et al. Perioperative strategies and technical modifications to the Nuss repair for pectus excavatum in pediatric patients: a large volume, single institution experience. J Pediatr Surg. 2014;49(4):575–82.
12. Kabbaj R, et al. Minimally invasive repair of pectus excavatum using the Nuss technique in children and adolescents: indications, outcomes, and limitations. Orthop Traumatol Surg Res. 2014;100(6):625–30.
13. Torre M, et al. Absorbable stabilisation of the bar in minimally invasive repair of pectus excavatum. Eur J Pediatr Surg. 2008;18(6):407–9.
14. Gürkök S, et al. The use of absorbable material in correction of pectus deformities. Eur J Cardiothorac Surg. 2001;19(5):711–2.
15. Kotzot D, Schwabegger AH. Etiology of chest wall deformities—a genetic review for the treating physician. J Pediatr Surg. 2009;44(10):2004–11.
16. Cobben JM, Oostra R-J, van Dijk FS. Pectus excavatum and carinatum. Eur J Med Genet. 2014;57(8):414–7.
17. Koumbourlis AC. Pectus excavatum: pathophysiology and clinical characteristics. Paediatr Respir Rev. 2009;10(1):3–6.
18. Goretsky MJ, Kelly Jr RE, Croitoru D, Nuss D. Chest wall anomalies: pectus excavatum and pectus carinatum. Adolesc Med Clin. 2004;15(3):455–71.
19. Obermeyer RJ, Goretsky MJ. Chest wall deformities in pediatric surgery. Surgical Clinics of North America. 2012;92(3):669–84.

Pectus Excavatum

4

Shyam K. Kolvekar and Nikolaos Panagiotopoulos

Abstract

Among all chest wall deformities Pectus Excavatum (PE) or funnel chest represents the most common congenital chest wall deformity accounting for 90 % of all deformities. The main characteristic is the depression of sternum and lower cartilages (Langer, Herrn JW Wiener med Zeit 49:515, 1880) with an incidence between 1 and 8 per 1000 children.

Keywords

Pectus Excavatum • Funnel chest • Congenital chest wall deformity

Pectus excavatum (PE) or funnel chest represents the most common congenital chest wall deformity accounting for 90 % of all deformities. Main characteristic is the depression of sternum and lower cartilages (Fig. 4.1, 4.2, and 4.3). The first description came from Bauhinus [1] in the sixteenth century. Another documented description of an appearance of the thorax could be found in 1860 by Woillez [2] and in 1863, von Luschka [3] reported about a 6-cm deep depression in the thorax wall of a 24-year-old man. Eggel [4] in 1870 published the first comprehensive case report of a patient with a funnel-formed thorax depression calling it a 'miraculum naturae'. He assumed that the reason for the deformity would be a weakness and an abnormal flexibility of the sternum caused by nutritional disturbance or by developmental failure. Individual case reports followed by Williams [5], Flesch [6] and Hagmann [7]. The latter believed that overgrowth of the ribs causes the depression of the chest. Langer and Zuckerkandel [8] favoured the hypothesis of a developmental failure, taking place in utero, in which the lower jaw of the foetus is responsible for the deformity by pushing on the sternum as a result of too high intrauterine pressure. Meyer performed the first operation of PE in 1911 with the removal of the rib cartilage [9]. He also analysed the removed cartilage microscopically and identified an unspecific degeneration.

The incidence of PE has a ratio between 1 and 8 per 1000 children [10]. Interestingly, males are more often affected, with a gender distribution

S.K. Kolvekar, MS, MCh, FRCS, FRCSCTh (✉)
Department of Cardiothoracic Surgery,
University College London Hospitals, The Heart Hospital and Barts Heart Center, London, UK
e-mail: kolvekar@yahoo.com

N. Panagiotopoulos, MD, PhD
Department of Cardiothoracic Surgery, University College London Hospitals (UCLH), London, UK

© Springer International Publishing Switzerland 2016
S.K. Kolvekar, H.K. Pilegaard (eds.), *Chest Wall Deformities and Corrective Procedures*,
DOI 10.1007/978-3-319-23968-2_4

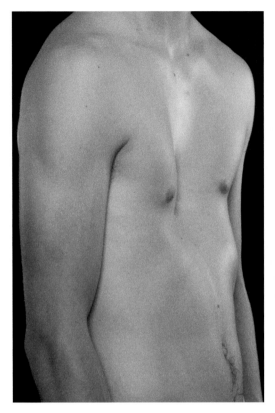

Fig. 4.1 Right side view in a 16-year-old

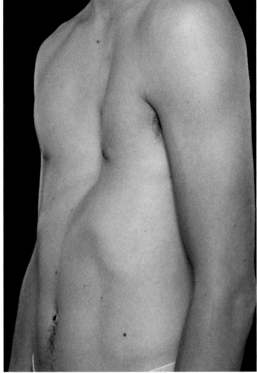

Fig. 4.2 Left side view in a 16-year-old

between 2:1 and 9:1 [11]. From the 19th century it has been recognised a genetic predisposition since a positive family history could be found in up to 43 % of PE cases [12, 13]. However, a specific genetic defect has not yet been found. Numerous syndromes are associated with PE and have been well described [14] where connective tissue disorder occurs in less than 1 % of all cases [15].

The majority of the patients with PE are tall, slim with associated scoliosis [14–16]. Severe depression of the sternum can cause displacement of the heart and reduction of lung volume [13, 17]. As a result of the anatomical changes, chest pain [12, 13, 15], fatigue [15], dyspnoea on exertion [12, 13, 15, 18], respiratory infections [13], asthma symptoms [13], palpitations [12] or heart murmurs could occur [13]. Several cases with mitral valve prolapse [13, 15, 19], mitral valve regurgitation and ventricle compression could be found [15, 17, 19]. For the latter, Coln [19] demonstrated that 95 % of 123 patients had cardiac compression. Even a single case report of syncopal symptoms has been

reported. The pulmonary and cardiovascular functions of patients with PE deformities were analysed in many investigations and have revealed measurable deficiencies [12]. Fonkalsrud [13] reported that the symptoms of many untreated PE patients become progressively worse with age and he recommended an operational intervention for both young and adult patients.

In contrast to these descriptions of more or less severe clinical signs, symptoms affecting daily life activities are either rare [20]. Therefore, some authors described the indication for a PE correction to be primarily cosmetic.

Numerous clinical studies described an improvement of pulmonary and/or cardiovascular symptoms and improvement in the subjective well-being after surgical correction [9, 13, 16–18]. Malek [18, 21] concluded that an operative intervention improves cardiovascular but not pulmonary function. Guntheroth [22] and Spiers as well as Johnson [23] re-evaluated the source data of Malek's meta-analyses and stated that due to

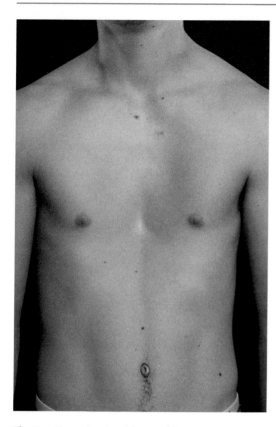

Fig. 4.3 Front view in a 16-year-old

relevant methodological deficits, these data failed to demonstrate any improvement of cardiac function. In this context, Aronson et al. [24] could not show an improvement in lung function parameters after Nuss procedure. Regardless the impact of the chest wall surgery to cardiopulmonary function the effect to psychological status of the patient is significant [15]. Numerous studies confirm that deformities cause relevant social discrimination, especially during adolescence, leading to the socio-psychologic problems [15]. A multicentre study demonstrated that the surgical repair of PE patients improves these socio-psychologic problems. [25–32]

References

1. Bauhinus J. Johannes Observatorium medicarum, rararum, novarum, admirabilium, et montrosarum, liber secundus. In: Ioannis Schenckii a Grafenberg, editor. Observation. Frankfurt: De partibus vitalibus, thorace contentis; 1609. p. 322.
2. Woillez. Sur un cas de deformitée thoracique considérable avec deplacement inoffensif de plusieur organes et signes sthetoscopiaques particulières. Paris: Rap Soc Med d'Hop; 1860. p. 3.
3. von Luschka H. Die Anatomie der Brust des Menschen. Die Anatomie des Menschen in Rücksicht auf die Bedürfnisse der praktischen Heilkunde. Tübingen: Laupp; 1863. p. 23
4. Eggel. Eine seltene Mißbildung des Thorax. Virchows Arch Path Anat. 1870;49:230.
5. Williams CT. Congenital malformation of the thorax great depression of the sternum. Trans Path Soc. 1872;24:50.
6. Flesch M. Über eine seltene Missbildung des Thorax. Virchows Arch Path Anat. 1873;75:289.
7. Hagmann. Selten vorkommende Abnormität des Brustkastens. Jb Kinderheilkunde. 1888;15:455.
8. Langer E. Zuckerkandel: Untersuchungen über den mißbildeten Brustkorb des. Herrn JW Wiener med Zeit. 1880;49:515.
9. Meyer L. Zur chirurgischen Behandlung der angeborenen Trichterbrust. Berl Klin Wschr. 1911;48:1563–6.
10. Kelly Jr RE, Lawson ML, Paidas CN, Hruban RH. Pectus excavatum in a 112-year autopsy series: anatomic findings and the effect on survival. J Pediatr Surg. 2005;40:1275–8.
11. Ravitch MM. Repair of pectus excavatum in children under 3 years of age: a twelve-year experience. Ann Thorac Surg. 1977;23:301.
12. Kelly Jr RE, Shamberger RC, Mellins RB, Mitchell KK, Lawson ML, Oldham K, et al. Prospective multicenter study of surgical correction of pectus excavatum: design, perioperative complications, pain, and baseline pulmonary function facilitated by internet-based data collection. J Am Coll Surg. 2007;205:205–16.
13. Fonkalsrud EW, Dunn JC, Atkinson JB. Repair of pectus excavatum deformities: 30 years of experience with 375 patients. Ann Surg. 2000;231:443–8.
14. Kotzot D, Schwabegger AH. Etiology of chest wall deformities—a genetic review for the treating physician. J Pediatr Surg. 2009;44:2004–11.
15. Colombani PM. Preoperative assessment of chest wall deformities. Semin Thorac Cardiovasc Surg. 2009;21:58–63.
16. Beiser GD, Epstein SE, Stampfer M, Goldstein RE, Noland SP, Levitsky S. Impairment of cardiac function in patients with pectus excavatum, with improvement after operative correction. N Engl J Med. 1972;287:267–72.
17. Kubiak R, Habelt S, Hammer J, Hacker FM, Mayr J, Bielek J. Pulmonary function following completion of Minimally Invasive Repair for Pectus Excavatum (MIRPE). Eur J Pediatr Surg. 2007;17:255–60.
18. Malek MH, Berger DE, Housh TJ, Marelich WD, Coburn JW, Beck TW. Cardiovascular function following surgical repair of pectus excavatum: a meta-analysis. Chest. 2006;130:506–16.

19. Coln E, Carrasco J, Coln D. Demonstrating relief of cardiac compression with the Nuss minimally invasive repair for pectus excavatum. J Pediatr Surg. 2006;41:683–6.
20. Luzzi L, Voltolini L, Zacharias J, Campione A, Ghiribelli C, Di Bisceglie M, et al. Ten year experience of bioabsorbable mesh support in pectus excavatum repair. Br J Plast Surg. 2004;57:733–40.
21. Malek MH, Berger DE, Marelich WD, Coburn JW, Beck TW, Housh TJ. Pulmonary function following surgical repair of pectus excavatum: a meta-analysis. Eur J Cardiothorac Surg. 2006;30:637–43.
22. Guntheroth WG, Spiers PS. Cardiac function before and after surgery for pectus excavatum. Am J Cardiol. 2007;99:1762–4.
23. Johnson JN, Hartman TK, Pianosi PT, Driscoll DJ. Cardiorespiratory function after operation for pectus excavatum. J Pediatr. 2008;153:359–64.
24. Aronson DC, Bosgraaf RP, Merz EM, van Steenwijk RP, van Aalderen WM, van Baren R. Lung function after the minimal invasive pectus excavatum repair (Nuss procedure). World J Surg. 2007;31:1518–22.
25. Kelly Jr RE, Cash TF, Shamberger RC, Mitchell KK, Mellins RB, Lawson ML, et al. Surgical repair of pectus excavatum markedly improves body image and perceived ability for physical activity: multicenter study. Pediatrics. 2008;122:1218–22.
26. Brown AL. Pectus excavatum (funnel chest). J Thorac Surg. 1939;9:164–84.
27. Sweet RH. Pectus excavatum: report of two cases successfully operated upon. Ann Surg. 1944;119:922–34.
28. Fokin AA, Robicsek F, Watts LT. Genetic analysis of connective tissue in patients with congenital thoracic abnormalities. Interact CardioVasc Thorac Surg. 2008;7:56.
29. Nakaoka T, Uemura S, Yano T, Nakagawa Y, Tanimoto T, Suehiro S. Does overgrowth of costal cartilage cause pectus excavatum? A study on the lengths of ribs and costal cartilages in asymmetric patients. J Pediatr Surg. 2009;44:1333–6.
30. Geisbe H, Buddecke E, Flach A, Muller G, Stein U. 88. Biochemical, morphological and physical as well as animal experimental studies on the pathogenesis of funnel chest. Langenbecks Arch Chir. 1967;319:536–41.
31. Rupprecht H, Hummer HP, Stoss H, Waldherr T. Pathogenesis of chest wall abnormalities—electron microscopy studies and trace element analysis of rib cartilage. Z Kinderchir. 1987;42:228–9.
32. Feng J, Hu T, Liu W, Zhang S, Tang Y, Chen R, et al. The biomechanical, morphologic, and histochemical properties of the costal cartilages in children with pectus excavatum. J Pediatr Surg. 2001;36:1770–6.

Pectus Carinatum

5

Shyam K. Kolvekar and Nikolaos Panagiotopoulos

Abstract

Pectus Carinatum (PC) or protrusion deformity of the chest wall accounts for 5 % of all chest wall deformities affecting 1 in 2500 live births (Ravitch, Congenital deformities of the chest wall and their operative correction. WB Saunders, Philadelphia, 1977). It is also know as pigeon chest. It can be unilateral, bilateral or mixed and there is predominance in males (Robicsek, Chest Surg Clin N Am 10(2):357–76, 2000).

Keywords

Pectus Carinatum • Pigeon chest • Congenital chest wall deformity

Pectus carinatum (PC) or protrusion deformity of the chest wall accounts for 5 % of all chest wall deformities affecting 1 in 2500 live births [1]. It can be unilateral, bilateral or mixed and there is predominance in males with a ration 4:1 [2]. However in some areas PC is almost equally or more frequent than PE [3, 4]. PC has not attributed the same interested as PE and the majority of the clinicians and thoracic surgeons are still unaware of surgical or conservative management options available. Since PC is rarely noticed at birth it is believed to be acquired rather than congenital. In most of cases it is perceived by the age of 10, is accentuated at puberty and reaches its peak at the ages of 16 and 18 respectively in female and male [3]. On the other hand a congenital association can be established by the following: presence at birth [4]; association with Marfan syndrome, congenital heart disease and hand agenesis [5]; observation in monozygotic twins [6, 7]; occurrence in more than two members in the same family. An association with reflux and mitral stenosis or prolapse has also been reported [8]. Another theory includes exaggerated growth of the cartilages [9, 10]. In PC an anterior growth can pull the sternum. Depending the location of the protrusion PC can be classified into the two following types:

- Inferior PC or chondrogladiolar (chicken breast or pigeon breast): It is the most frequent

S.K. Kolvekar, MS, MCh, FRCS, FRCSCTh (✉)
Department of Cardiothoracic Surgery,
University College London Hospitals, The Heart Hospital and Barts Heart Center, London, UK
e-mail: kolvekar@yahoo.com

N. Panagiotopoulos, MD, PhD
Department of Cardiothoracic Surgery, University College London Hospitals (UCLH), London, UK

type and characterize by a prominent sternum mainly in its mid and lower portion. In almost all cases is associated with lower bilateral costal depression. It is more often symmetric (Figs. 5.1, 5.2, and 5.3).

• Superior PC or chondromanubrium (pouter pigeon or Currarino & Silverman syndrome): It consists of upper protrusion of the sternal

notch that is proximal to midsternum and lower pseudo depression. It is subdivided to upper PC with midsternum depression and without midsternuml depression [11].

Clinically the deformity presents a typical progressive growth and can be accompanied by cardiovascular and respiratory symptoms similar

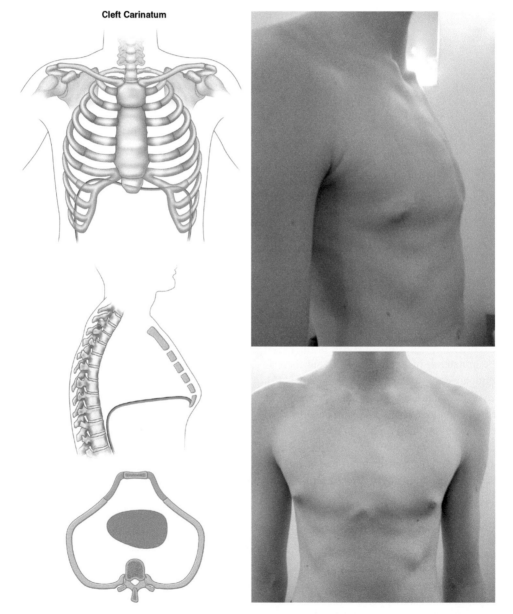

Figs. 5.1, 5.2, and 5.3 Inferior PC or chondrogladiolar (chicken breast or pigeon breast): It is the most frequent type and characterize by a prominent sternum mainly in its mid and lower portion. In almost all cases is associated with lower bilateral costal depression. It is more often symmetric

to PE. These usually include palpitations, dyspnoea, wheezing with exertion and reduced exercise tolerance. Usually the cardiac and pulmonary function are less implicated than in PE but psychological effects of PC can be severe and responsible for low self esteem [12] leading to the necessity of a surgical correction.

References

1. Nuss D, Croitoru DP, Kelly RE. Congenital chest wall deformities. In: Ashcraft KW, Holcomb III GW, Murphy JP, editors. Pediatric surgery. 4th ed. Philadelphia: Elsevier Saunders; 2005. p. 245–63.
2. Shamberger RC, Welch KJ. Surgical correction of pectus carinatum. J Pediatr Surg. 1987;22:48–53.
3. Acastello E. Patologias de la pared toracica en pediatria. Buenos Aires: Editorial El Ateneo; 2006.
4. Martinez-Ferro M, Fraire C, Bernard S. Dynamic compression system for the correction of pectus carinatum. Semin Pediatr Surg. 2008;17(3):194–200.
5. Lodi R, Bondioli A, Curti L, Bruni GC, Palmieri B. Surgical correction of the pectus excavatum and carinatum in the adult. Report of an unusual case of combination of the straight back and pectus excavatum. Minerva Chir. 1975;30(3):131–8.
6. Currarino G, Silverman FN. Premature obliteration of sternal suture and pigeon-breast deformity. Radiology. 1958;70(4):532–40.
7. Lam CR, Taber RE. Surgical treatment of pectus carinatum. Arch Surg. 1971;103(2):191–4.
8. Chidambaram B, Mehta AV. Currarino-Silverman syndrome (pectus carinatum type 2 deformity) and mitral valve disease. Chest. 1992;102(3):780–2.
9. Lester CW. Pigeon breast (pectus carinatum) and other protrusion deformities of the chest of developmental origin. Ann Surg. 1953;137(4):482–9.
10. Ravitch MM. Congenital deformities of the chest wall and their operative correction. Philadelphia: WB Saunders; 1977.
11. Robicsek F. Surgical treatment of pectus carinatum. Chest Surg Clin N Am. 2000;10(2):357–76.
12. Fonkalsrud EW, Anselmo DM. Less extensive techniques for repair of pectus carinatum: the undertreated chest deformity. J Am Coll Surg. 2004;198(6):898–905.

Investigations for Chest Wall Deformities

Rajeev Shukla, Trupti Kolvekar, and Shyam K. Kolvekar

Abstract

Congenital chest wall deformities encompass a wide spectrum of conditions and present the patient with varying severities of cardiorespiratory and psychological dysfunction. Surgical intervention has been shown to alleviate symptoms and improve overall psychological wellbeing. Throughout history many different surgical correction techniques have been described for the treatment of congenital chest deformities. One factor that is common to all these surgical techniques is the necessity for detailed pre-operative workup. This chapter aims to explore the imaging modalities that can be used in the pre-operative evaluation of patients with a spectrum of congenital chest wall deformities.

Keywords

Pectus excavatum • Funnel chest • Haller Index • Nuss • Imaging • MRI • Chest x-ray • CMR • Sternal imaging • Jeune Syndrome • Asphyxiating thoracic dystrophy • Poland Syndrome • Sternal cleft

R. Shukla, MChem(Hons), MB, BS(Lon)
Department of Cardiothoracic Surgery, The Heart Hospital, University College London Hospital NHS Trust, London, UK

T. Kolvekar, BSc Biochemistry (Hon)
The Department of Structural Molecular Biology, University College London, London, UK

S.K. Kolvekar, MS, MCh, FRCS, FRCS (CTh) (✉)
Department of Cardiothoracic Surgery, University College London Hospitals, The Heart Hospital and Barts Heart Center, London, UK
e-mail: kolvekar@yahoo.com

Introduction

Pectus excavatum (PE) is the most common congenital chest deformity. It is characterised by posterior depression of the sternum and adjacent costal cartilages, thereby reducing the antero-posterior distance of the thoracic cage [1, 2]. As many as 50 % of patients have a right sided dominant sternal depression [3]. Most patients present in their first year of life, but rarely do infants and young children exhibit clinical symptoms [4]. In adolescence patients may present

© Springer International Publishing Switzerland 2016
S.K. Kolvekar, H.K. Pilegaard (eds.), *Chest Wall Deformities and Corrective Procedures*,
DOI 10.1007/978-3-319-23968-2_6

with cardiorespiratory symptoms, including exercise intolerance, fatigue, decreased stamina, exercise-induced wheezing [3, 4]. As many as 25 % of PE patients have increased incidence of respiratory tract infections or asthma and more than 50 % experience sharp pains in the lower anterior chest. Tachypnoea and palpitations are also common [3].

Moderate to severe deformities can result in significant displacement of the heart into the left chest resulting in considerable physiological impairment. Compression of the heart between the sternum and vertebral column was evident in early pathological studies [5] and thus explain some of the symptoms experienced by patients.

Throughout history many surgical correction techniques for PE have been described. One factor that is common to all these surgical techniques is the necessity for detailed pre-operative workup subsequent to patient selection for operative intervention [6]. This section explores the variety of imaging modalities that can be effectively utilised in evaluating the severity of PE and thus a means for quantifying the deformity.

Haller Index

Imaging for detailed anatomical assessment of PE deformity forms an essential component of preoperative workup and enables accurate quantification of the severity of sternal depression, the Haller Index [7].

The Haller Index was developed from CT scan analysis of a single image of the deepest part of the PE deformity. In their study Haller et al. calculated the ratio between the transverse diameter and the anteroposterior diameter, measured from the posterior surface of the sternum to the anterior surface of the vertebral body at the point of maximal depression. This was performed in 33 patients who underwent corrective surgery for PE deformity and compared with age-matched nonpectus controls. Haller found that all operated patients had a Haller Index of >3.25 (mean 4.42) and non-pectus controls <3.25 (mean 2.56) [8–11]. In adolescents and children, the Haller

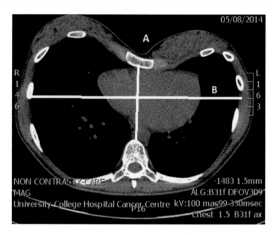

Fig. 6.1 Haller Index on CT scan

Index may range from 1.9 to 2.7 due to differences in chest wall configuration linked to age and gender. It was found that girls between ages 0–6 years and 12–18 years tended to have a higher Haller index than boys of the same age [12–15]. In clinical practice, it is widely accepted that a Haller Index >3.25 is indicative of a severe pectus deformity [16]. When combined with criteria obtained from adjunct tests including pulmonary function tests, cardiology evaluation to determine cardiovascular physiological impairment, a Haller Index >3.25 can be an indication for surgical correction [2, 8, 10, 11]. Various imaging modalities have been employed during the evaluation of pectus deformity with the aim to provide an accurate Haller Index and additional information regarding the effects on the local anatomy (Fig. 6.1) [2, 13, 14].

Chest X-ray

Evaluation of patients with plain radiographs is performed in two projections, frontal and lateral [15, 16]. PE deformity can produce characteristic findings of right middle lobe opacification on the frontal view that can often be mistaken for right middle lobe pneumonia or atelectasis [15]. This abnormal appearance is in fact due to compression of anterior chest wall soft tissue [15]. Other features that may also be apparent on frontal

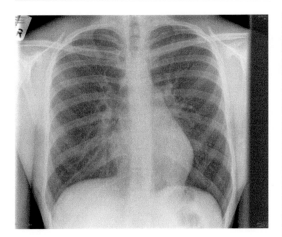

Fig. 6.2 Chest x-ray PA view

projections include displacement of the cardiac silhouette to the left in more than 50 % of patients [17]. Takahashi et al. found obliteration of the descending aortic interface in 30 % of PE cases reviewed retrospectively in a cohort of 70 patients. Although no significant relationship was found between this and the severity of thoracic deformity, an indirect correlation to cardiac rotation angle does appear evident [18].

Lateral projections demonstrate posterior displacement of the sternum that is evident as an opacity filling the retrosternal space with ribs projecting anterior to the sternum, thus confirming PE deformity (Figs. 6.2, 6.3, 6.4, and 6.5) [15].

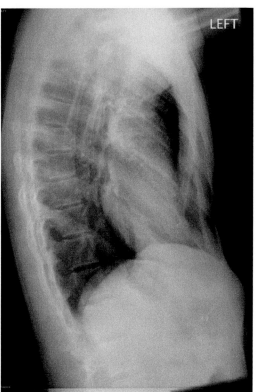

Fig. 6.3 Chest x-ray with left lateral view

CT Scan

Computerised tomography (CT) scans have long been the primary imaging modality for evaluation of PE deformity. As described earlier, the Haller Index for objectively grading the severity of PE deformity was developed through the use of CT scans by dividing the transverse diameter of the chest by the anteroposterior diameter at the point of maximal sternal depression. In addition, CT scans can effectively demonstrate the degree of cardiac compression and displacement and its relationship to the sternum, the degree of pulmonary compression and atelectasis, asymmetry of the chest, sternal torsion and compensatory

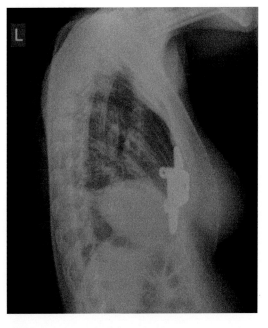

Fig. 6.4 Chest x-ray left lateral with the bar

development of a barrel chest (Figs. 6.6, 6.7, 6.8, 6.9, 6.10, and 6.11) [2, 19].

rotation, great vessel anomalies and asymmetric volume between left and right hemithorax (Fig. 6.12) [20, 21].

MRI and CMR

Certain centres have adopted Magnetic Resonance Imaging as the primary imaging modality to calculate the Haller Index. The primary advantage over CT is the absence of ionising radiation [10]. Piccolo et al. demonstrated strong comparability of Haller Indices and Asymmetry Indices obtained using fast MRI and CT scanning. In addition, fast MRI demonstrates excellent soft tissue contrast and thus high quality assessment of cardiac displacement or

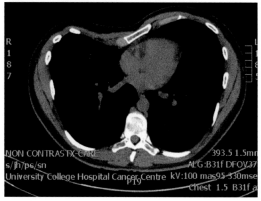

Fig. 6.7 CT scan with tilt of sternum with depressed right side

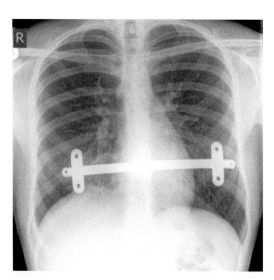

Fig. 6.5 Chest x-ray with the bar

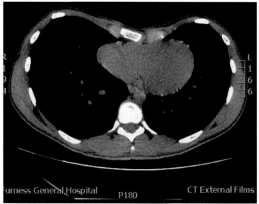

Fig. 6.8 CT scan with depression more on left side

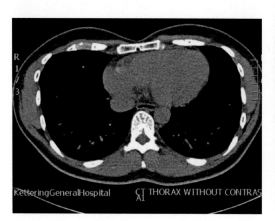

Fig. 6.6 CT scan with minimal depression and displacement

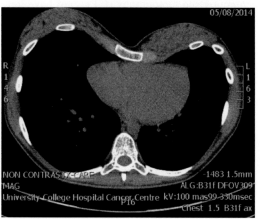

Fig. 6.9 CT scan with leftward tilt and depression

Fig. 6.10 3D reconstruction from CT showing the sternal depression and ribs alignment (**a**) lateral view; (**b**) oblique view

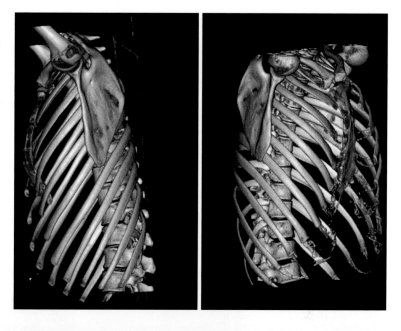

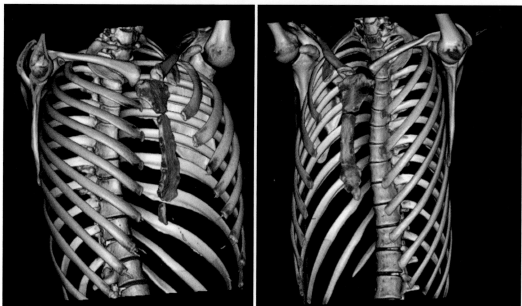

Fig. 6.11 3D reconstruction from CT showing the sternal depression and ribs alignment oblique view (**a**) right oblique view; (**b**) left oblique view

CMR has also been investigated as a potential imaging modality with the aim to delineate the anatomical and physiological components of pectus excavatum in addition to calculating the Haller Index. Saleh et al. demonstrated statistically significant higher HI in PE patients compared to non pectus patients (9.6 versus 2.8). The group were also able to demonstrate significant left lateral shift of the heart compared to controls (84 % versus 64 %) and reduction in right ventricular ejection fraction, which may be suggestive of changes in myocardial performance [22]. Humphries et al. have also demonstrated similar results with calculated HI of PE and non pectus patients [23].

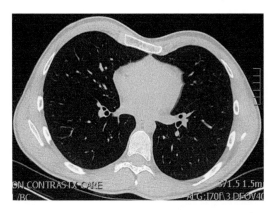

Fig. 6.12 MRI scan transverse section showing sternal depression

Echocardiography

Echocardiograms are performed to search for the presence of major valvular pathology and chamber compression (Fig. 6.13). The right ventricle and atrium can be compressed by the sternum resulting in problems during diastolic filling [20].

Mitral valve prolapse is seen in up to 17 % of patients with PE. Evaluation of the aortic root is also important particularly in patients who have been diagnosed with Marfans Syndrome [3, 7, 20].

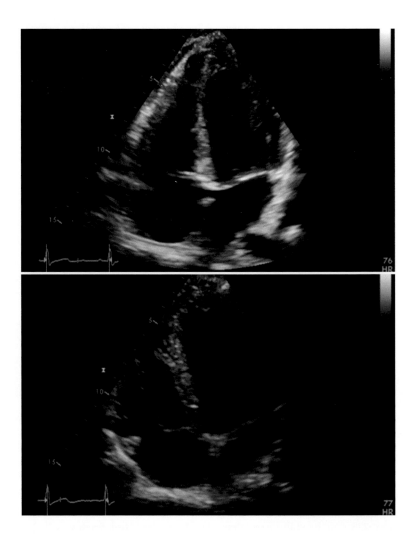

Fig. 6.13 Echocardiogram with four-channel view

Summary

Recent discussion has questioned the absolute necessity of performing a CT scan for evaluation of PE deformity. The main factor in searching for alternative imaging techniques is the high doses of radiation that are being delivered by CT scans to patients in their adolescence or younger who are being assessed for PE deformity. Four independent groups have evaluated the use of two-view chest x-rays in the pre-operative assessment of patients with PE deformity and conclude strong comparability of HI calculated from chest x-rays with that of CT scans and strong interobserver correlation. The unanimous recommendations from these studies is to replace CT imaging with chest X rays as the primary imaging modality for PE surgical workup, which would result in a 100 fold reduction in effective radiation dose [1, 24–26]. The counter argument to this is that chest x-rays provide no information regarding sternal asymmetry or torsion or the degree of cardiac compression and displacement [19]. One study concluded that no additional information was gleaned from a CT scan that was not already evident from two-view CXRs and instead adopted the use of low dose CT scanning comprising of five to seven slices through the point of maximal sternal depression in addition to two view CXRs. This has reduced radiation doses by up to 80 % [27] while still providing comprehensive visualisation of the local anatomy. In addition to significantly reducing the radiation exposure a substantial cost saving is also achievable when employing this strategy for pre-operative assessment [24].

Other groups have investigated the use of MRI and CMR scanning as the primary imaging modality and thus eliminating ionising radiation exposure completely. Two separate studies have shown favourable results for using MRI over CT scans to calculate the HI and AI while detailing anatomical information such as displacement, rotation or compression of the heart or great vessel anomalies [10, 21]. In addition to no radiation exposure the images can be acquired in less than 5 min without any compromise in quality. Further research demonstrates that cine MR can provide additional diagnostic information through evaluation of chest morphology and chest wall kinetics [10]. CMR has also been shown to be beneficial for the same reasons as MRI but also in its ability to provide accurate and dynamic assessment of cardiovascular function and thus potentially eliminating the need for echocardiographic studies.

It is clear that a growing number of institutions are moving away from the use of full chest CT scanning as the primary modality for calculating HI and AI in patients with PE deformity and adopting imaging strategies that have lower or no radiation exposure. All of the studies performed with alternative imaging modalities to CT have a smaller cohort of patients but so far the results are encouraging.

Pectus Carinatum

Pectus carinatum (PC) is the second most common anterior chest wall anomaly occurring in approximately one in 1500 live births with a male to female ratio of 4:1 [20, 28]. It is characterised by sternal and costal cartilage elevation [20] and depending on the area involved can be classified into two variant types [20, 28].

Chondrogladiolar subtype is the more common deformity involving protrusion of the mid to lower portion of the anterior chest wall and inferior costal cartilages and part of the gladiolus [28, 29]. Chondromanubrial deformity or Currarino-Silverman syndrome in cases with associated congenital heart disease, is the less common subtype involving protrusion of the second and third costal cartilages with elevation of the sterno-manubrial joint [20, 28].

Pre-treatment radiological evaluation of PC aims to establish the presence of an increased antero-posterior (AP) diameter in association with protrusion of the sternum [28]. Features that may be apparent on plain chest radiography

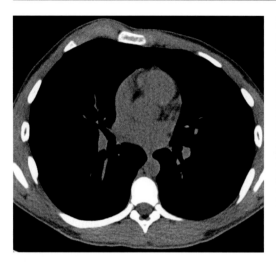

Fig. 6.14 Uneven shape

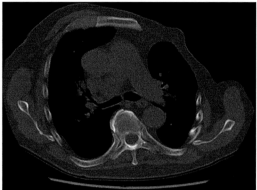

Fig. 6.15 CT scan with left sided hypoplasia

include a narrowed thorax and scoliosis on posteroanterior projections. Lateral projections provide a more striking image of the deformity. Features that can be identified include the presence of a bowed, short, comma-shaped sternum with an increased AP diameter [28]. Further differentiation of PC into its variant forms, as determined by the site of sternal protrusion, can also be adequately demonstrated on lateral projections as shown by various groups [28–31]. Computed tomography (CT) has also been advocated for use in the evaluation of patients with PC as part of the routine pre-treatment assessment (Fig. 6.14) [20]. Desmaris et al. conclude that CT scanning should be reserved for cases with 'mixed' deformities, where sternal angle measurements can be easily calculated [30]. More recently Lee et al. presented their experience with the use of MRI for evaluation of PC. Early results show MRI to be highly effective at measuring sternal angle rotation and asymmetry index in PC patients, which can be used in pre-treatment evaluations [32].

Poland Syndrome

Poland syndrome (PS) is an uncommon chondrocostal anomaly occurring in approximately 1 in 30,000 live births [33, 34]. It is characterised by

the absence or hypoplasia of the costosternal part of the pectoralis major and minor muscle and absent costal cartilages or ribs 2, 3 and 4 or 3, 4 and 5 [33–35]. PS is essentially a unilateral defect and may be associated with lung herniation. Two-thirds of cases involve the right side [34, 35]. Surgical intervention in PS is reconstructive to protect organs, which are at risk of damage due to bony defects and cosmetic to fill the defect resulting from absent pectoralis muscles [20]. The primary imaging modalities used in pre-operative assessment include chest radiography and computed tomography (CT) (Fig. 6.15) [20, 33]. Unilateral hyperlucency mimicking radical mastectomy is often seen in chest radiography [33]. However, for detailed assessment of the extent of muscular, rib and costal cartilage involvement a combined imaging using CT and MRI has been advocated, with CT providing a clearer depiction of bony defects and the absence of the pectoralis minor muscle and MRI providing better tissue contrast [36]. CT scan with 3D reconstruction allows for greater anatomical detail thereby enhancing surgical planning [20, 36, 37].

Sternal Cleft

A sternal cleft is a rare abnormality, which is classified as partial or complete. Partial defects can be located superiorly or inferiorly. Complete defects arise as a result of complete lack of fusion of the sternum in the midline [28, 34].

CT is considered to be the imaging modality of choice as it depicts midline defects clearly and when reformatted can delineate between complete and incomplete defects [28]. Successful prenatal diagnosis of sternal clefts using 3D and 4D sonography have been reported by various groups [6, 38, 39]. Pasoglou et al. [39] reported a multimodality approach to imaging of sternal cleft using CT, MRI and US. The latter investigations can be used prenataly without exposing the foetus to radiation. However, images obtained by US can be affected by maternal obesity [40]. CT is recommended for use in the neonatal period to safely exclude the presence of associated skeletal abnormalities [39].

Jeune Syndrome

Jeune syndrome [asphyxiating thoracic dystrophy (ATD)] is a rare autosomal recessive genetic disorder causing skeletal dysplasia [41, 42]. It is characterised by a small, narrow thoracic cage and variable limb shortness [41, 43]. Radiographic findings are specific enough to enable easy distinction from other skeletal dysplasias except the Ellis-van Crevald syndrome [41, 44]. Typical findings include a narrow, bell-shaped thorax with short, horizontal orientation of ribs and irregular costochondral junctions, elevated clavicles, short iliac bones with a typical trident appearance of the acetabula, relatively short and wide long bones of the extremeties and hypoplastic phalanges of both hands and feet with cone-shaped epiphyses [41, 42]. Various groups report the value of performing prenatal sonography in diagnosing a foetus with severe forms of ATD. The important findings suggestive of a diagnosis of ATD included severe shortened ribs, thorax, short limbs without polydactyl [45–47].

References

1. Wu T-H, et al. Usefulness of chest images for the assessment of pectus excavatum before and after a Nuss repair in adults. Eur J Cardiothorac Surg. 2013;43:283–7.
2. Frantz FW. Indications and guidelines for pectus excavatum repair. Curr Opin Pediatr. 2011;23:486–91.
3. Fonkalsrud EW. Current management of pectus excavatum. World J Surg. 2003;27:502–8.
4. Sawar ZU, DeFlorio R, O'Connor SC. Pectus excavatum: current imaging techniques and opportunities for dose reduction. Semin Ultrasound CT MR. 2014;35(4):374–81.
5. Malek MH, et al. Cardiovascular function following surgical repair of pectus excavatum – a metaanalysis. Chest. 2006;130:506–16.
6. Brochhausen C, et al. Pectus excavatum: history, hypotheses and treatment options. Interact Cardiovasc Thorac Surg. 2012;14:801–6.
7. Jaroszewski D, Notrica D, McMahon L, Steidley ED, Deschamps C. Current management of pectus excavatum: a review and update of therapy and treatment recommendations. J Am Board Fam Med. 2010;23:230–9.
8. Haller AJ, Kramer SS, Lietman SA. Use of CT scans in selection of patients for pectus excavatum surgery: a preliminary report. J Pediatr Surg. 1987;22(10):904–6.
9. Rebeis EB, et al. Anthropometric index for quantitative assessment of pectus excavatum. J Bras Pneumol. 2004;30(6):501–7.
10. Marcovici PA, LoSasso BE, Kruk P, Dwek JR. MRI for the evaluation of pectus excavatum. Pediatr Radiol. 2011;41:757–8.
11. Blanco FC, Elliott ST, Sandler AD. Chest wall reconstruction. Semin Plast Surg. 2011;25:107–16.
12. Eich GF, Kellenberg CJ, Willi UV. Radiology of the chest wall. Paediatric chest imaging: chest imaging in infants and children. Springer, Berlin. 2013; p. 315–6.
13. Nuss D, Kelly RE. Indications and technique of Nuss procedure for pectus excavatum. Thorac Surg Clin. 2010;20:583–97.
14. Kelly RE. Pectus excavatum: historical background, pre-operative evaluation and criteria for operation. Semin Pediatr Surg. 2008;17(3):181–93.
15. Robbins LP. Pectus excavatum. Radiol Case Rep (online). 2011;6:460.
16. Baez JC, Lee EY, Restrepo R, Eisenberg RL. Chest wall lesions in children. AJR Am J Roentgenol. 2013;200:W402–19.
17. Morshuis WJ, et al. Chest radiography in pectus excavatum: recognition of pectus excavatum-related signs and assessment of severity before and after surgical correction. Eur Radiol. 1994;4(3):197–202.
18. Takahashi K, Sugimoto H, Ohsawa T. Obliteration of the descending aortic interface in pectus excavatum: correlation with clockwise rotation of the heart. Radiology. 1992;182(3):825–8.
19. Goretsky MJ, Kelly RE, Croitoru D, Nuss D. Chest wall anomalies: pectus excavatum and pectus carinatum. Adolesc Med. 2004;15:455–71.
20. Colombani P. Preoperative assessment of chest wall deformities. Semin Thorac Cardiovasc Surg. 2009;21:58–63.
21. Piccolo RL, et al. Chest fast MRI: an imaging alternative on pre-operative evaluation of pectus excavatum. J Pediatr Surg. 2012;47:485–9.

22. Saleh RS, et al. Cardiovascular magnetic resonance in patients with pectus excavatum compared with normal controls. J Cardiovasc Magn Reson. 2010;12:73. 1–10.

23. Humprhies CM, Anderson JL, Flores JH, Doty JR. Cardiac magnetic resonance imaging for perioperative evaluation of sternal eversion for pectus excavatum. Eur J Cardiothorac Surg. 2013;43:1110–3.

24. Poston PM, et al. Defining the role of chest radiography in determining candidacy for pectus excavatum repair. Innovations. 2014;9(2):117–21.

25. Khanna G, Jaju A, Don S, Keys T, Hildebolt CF. Comparison of Haller Index values calculated with chest radiographs versus CT for pectus excavatum evaluation. Pediatr Radiol. 2010;40:1763–7.

26. Mueller C, Saint-Vil D, Bouchard S. Chest x-ray as a primary modality for preoperative imaging of pectus excavatum. J Pediatr Surg. 2008;43:71–3.

27. Rattan AS, Laor T, Ryckman FC, Brody AS. Pectus excavatum imaging: enough but not too much. Pediatr Radiol. 2010;40:168–72.

28. Restrepo CS, et al. Imaging appearances of the sternum and sternoclavicular joints. Radiographics. 2009;29:839–59.

29. Shamberger RC, Welch KJ. Surgical correction of pectus carinatum. J Pediatr Surg. 1987;22(1):48–53.

30. Desmaris TJ, Keller M. Pectus carinatum. Curr Opin Pediatr. 2013;25(3):375–81.

31. Grissom LE, Harcke HT. Thoracic deformities and the growing lung. Semin Roentgenol. 1998;33(2):199–208.

32. Lee R, et al. MRI evaluation of pectus carinatum: preliminary experience. European Congress of Radiology. Scientific Exhibit Poster, Vienna C-0022; 2015.

33. Jeung MY, et al. Imaging of chest wall disorders. Radiographics. 1999;19:617–37.

34. Torre et al. Chest wall deformities: an overview on classification and surgical options, chap. 8. In: Topics in thoracic surgery. InTech, Europe. 2012. p. 117–36.

35. Urschel Jr HC. Poland syndrome. Semin Thorac Cardiovasc Surg. 2009;21(1):89–94.

36. Ribeiro RC, et al. Clinical and radiographic poland syndrome classification: a proposal. Aesthet Surg J. 2009;29(6):494–504.

37. Cingel V, et al. Poland syndrome: from embryological basis to plastic surgery. Surg Radiol Anat. 2013;35(8):639–46.

38. Izquierdo MT, Bahamonde A, Domene J. Prenatal diagnosis of a complete cleft sternum with 3-dimensional sonography. J Ultrasound Med. 2009;28:379–83.

39. Pasoglou V, et al. Sternal cleft: prenatal multimodality imaging. Pediatr Radiol. 2012;42:1014–6.

40. Twomey EL, et al. Prenatal ultrasonography and neonatal imaging of complete cleft sternum: a case report. Ultrasound Obstet Gynecol. 2005;25:599–601.

41. Thakkar PA, Aiyer S, Shah B. Asphyxiating thoracic dystrophy (Jeune syndrome). J Case Rep. 2012;2(1):15–7.

42. de Vries J, et al. Jeune syndrome: description of 13 cases and a proposal for follow-up protocol. Eur J Pediatr. 2010;169(1):77–88.

43. Shaheen R, et al. A founder CEP120 mutation in Jeune asphyxiating thoracic dystrophy expands the role of centriolar proteins in skeletal ciliopathies. Hum Mol Genet. 2015;24(5):1410–9.

44. Oberklaid F, et al. Asphyxiating thoracic dysplasia. Clinical, radiological and pathological information on 10 patients. Arch Dis Child. 1977;52(10):758–65.

45. Tongsong T, et al. Prenatal sonographic findings associated with asphyxiating thoracic dystrophy (Jeune syndrome). J Ultrasound Med. 1999;18:573–6.

46. Hollander NS, et al. Early prenatal sonographic diagnosis and follow-up of Jeune syndrome. Ultrasound Obstet Gynecol. 2001;18:378–83.

47. Schinzel A, et al. Prenatal sonographic diagnosis of Jeune syndrome. Radiology. 1985;154(3):777–8.

Indexes for Pectus Deformities

7

Marcelo Martinez-Ferro

Abstract

A thoracic index is a formula used to qualify or quantify a thoracic deformity and in some cases, to define strategies within treatment. It is also a diagnostic tool used historically to assess the severity of the defect. There is no definition, classification, or consensus in the literature on which thoracic index is the gold standard. There are also no guidelines regarding cut-off values. This chapter is an effort to put all this together, starting by defining thoracic indexes, proposing a classification and describing them in detail for the first time. The main objective is to find out which are the most commonly indexes used by chest wall malformation experts worldwide, and why. For this reason the present chapter includes a web-based survey made to the aforementioned experts in order to review this issue in detail. Since there is currently no thoracic index without limitations, perhaps the perfect index is a mathematical combination of several different indexes. Perhaps it is one single index still to be discovered. This is the first step to search for a universal thoracic index for surgical – decision making.

Keywords

Thoracic Index • Haller Index • Pectus Excavatum • Severity • Surgery

Introduction

There is presently no definition of "thoracic index" or consensus in the literature on which one is the gold standard. There are also no

M. Martinez-Ferro, MD
Department of Surgery, Fundacion Hospitalaria
Children's Hospital, Buenos Aires, Argentina
e-mail: m.martinezferro@gmail.com

guidelines regarding cut-off values. Assessment of patients and the process of surgical-decision making vary considerably among chest wall malformations experts worldwide [1–3]. Moreover, even though thoracic indexes can be used to evaluate any chest wall malformation they are commonly employed to study Pectus Excavatum (PE) patients. The objective of this chapter is to review this topic and to report the results and observations from a web-based survey.

© Springer International Publishing Switzerland 2016
S.K. Kolvekar, H.K. Pilegaard (eds.), *Chest Wall Deformities and Corrective Procedures*,
DOI 10.1007/978-3-319-23968-2_7

Definition

Basically a thoracic index is formula employed to characterize a set of data obtained from thoracic (basically anterior chest wall and cardiac) measurements. It is a diagnostic tool used historically to assess the severity of the deformity. A thoracic index comprises a cut-off point, that is, a limit at which expectant treatment for a pathology, as PE, is or is not longer applicable. Additionally, it allows surgeons to define strategies within treatment. Thoracic indexes vary with age, gender, body mass, and morphology (cup, saucer, grand canyon, and other shape depressions), among other factors [2–7].

Usefulness of Thoracic Indexes

1. To assess the severity of the defect
2. To establish a cut-off point for treatment indication
3. To define treatment strategies
4. To quantify postoperative changes in the shape of the chest

Recent thoracic indexes have been focused not only on the severity of the defect as aforementioned, but on characteristics of the sternum, the deformity, and the impact PE has on the patients' cardiopulmonary function [8, 9].

Type of Thoracic Indexes

Diagnostic Indexes
1. Clinical Indexes
2. Chest-X-Ray Indexes
3. Chest-CT-Scan Indexes
4. Chest and Cardiac MRI Indexes
5. Other Indexes

Subtype of Thoracic Indexes

Assessment Indexes
1. Sternal Indexes
2. Severity Indexes

3. Deformity Indexes
4. Cardiac Indexes

Classification

There is presently no classification of thoracic indexes. In an effort to organize the large amount of diagnostic and assessment indexes in existence until date, the following classification is proposed (Table 7.1).

It must be pointed out however that, even though cardio-pulmonary function tests are rarely indicated for surgical decision making, evaluation of the impact of the sternal depression on the lung and heart are helpful for achieve a full diagnosis of the defect, deal with health insurance companies and enable the patient and family understand that the PE is not only an aesthetic problem.

Validation

Validation is the confirmation of the experience or judgment of one author by another and is achieved by repeating another author's work and reaching the same results. The same materials, methods, inclusion and exclusion criteria have to be used. Publishing the validated results is encouraged to reinforce the author's original experience and findings. The Haller Index cut-off point of 3.25 used for surgical indication, for example, has never been validated by other authors, even though a great deal of chest wall malformation experts use it routinely in their practice. Although a huge variety of indexes have been described in the literature, only few authors have validated some of them. An example of validation is the recent publication of Poston et. al. in which the Correction Index described by St. Peter et al. was analyzed obtaining similar results than those obtained by the original authors.

Description

The most frequently reported thoracic indexes will be hereby described.

Table 7.1 Proposed classification of the most commonly reported thoracic indexes

Type	Subtype	Thoracic indexes
Diagnostic indexes	Assessment indexes	Most commonly reported indexes
Clinical		Anthropometric Index [5, 10–12]
Chest X-ray	Sternal	Vertebral Index [7, 10, 13–16]
		Welch Index [17, 18]
		Haje Body Manubrial Index [2]
		Haje Body Manubrial Xyphoid Index [2]
	Severity	Chest-X-Ray Haller Index [19–21]
	Deformity	Configuration Index [7]
		Frontosagittal Index [16]
Chest CT scan	Sternal	Haje Width Length Index [1]
	Severity	Haller Index [22–24]
		Modified Haller Index In expiration [24, 25] For carinatum [7]
		Correction Index [19, 26]
	Deformity	Asymmetry Index [6, 27–29]
		Vertebral Index [28]
		Frontosagittal Index [28]
		Steepness Index [27]
		Excavatum Volume Index [27]
		Depression Index [28, 30]
		Eccentricity Index [28, 29]
		Unbalance Index [28]
		Flatness Index [29]
		Circularity Index [29]
	Cardiac	Cardiac Compression Index [31]
		Cardiac Asymmetry Index [31]
		Modified Cardiac Compression Index [24]
Chest and cardiac MRI	Sternal, severity, deformity and cardiac	All the aforementioned
		Cardiac MRI Indexes [32–37, 45]
Other[a]		Stress cardiac ultrasound [38]
		Pletismography [39]
		External body scanner Indexes [38, 40]

[a]These thoracic indexes will not be assessed in the current chapter

Clinical Indexes

Anthropometric Index

As stated by its authors, the **Anthropometric Index (AI)** is a quickly administered and low-cost clinical assessment tool, which does not induce any adverse effects and is not vulnerable to environmental influences. The A and B clinical measurements are carried out with the patient in a horizontal supine position on a flat table parallel to the floor during deep inhalation. The A measurement is defined as the largest antero-posterior diameter at the level of the distal third of the sternum, and the B measurement, as the largest depth at the same level.

The AI for PE is calculated by dividing B by A (Fig. 7.1) [5]. The AI cut-off point for PE pre- and postoperatively is 0.12.

Anthropometric Index = B/A

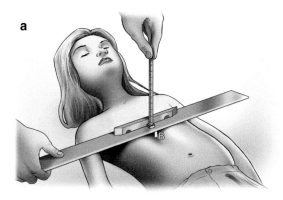

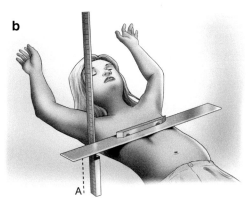

Fig. 7.1 Schematic representation of a PE patient for the calculation of the **Anthropometric Index**. (**a**) measurement of the anteroposterior distance during deep inhalation at the distal third of the sternum. (**b**) measurement during deep inhalation at the greater depth, at the distal third of the sternum. The instruments used were: an articulated square, a rigid ruler coupled to a level (the measuring device), a pinned limiting device and a conventional ruler

The case series presented by Rebeis et al. [10] exhibited significant difference between male and female patients. The authors believed that the breasts accounted for this difference because measurements A and B were obtained using gauging devices that run across the chest. This belief is supported by no difference being found between male and female preteen subjects (3–10 years), when the breasts have not yet been developed. Authors such as Knutson [11] and Horst et al. [12] endorse the AI.

Chest X-ray Indexes

Because direct measurements are subject to variations in age, height, and body mass, radiographic indexes were also developed.

Vertebral Index

Authors such as Rebeis et al. [10], Welch [17], Backer et al. [13], Hummer and Willital [15], Haller et al. [22], and Derveaux et al. [7] formulated individual indexes to quantify the severity of the deformity and/or to enable the comparison between preoperative and postoperative results more objectively. All of them have in common that their indexes relate the approximation of the sternum to the spinal column. The Vertebral Index (**VI**) is calculated from a lateral thoracic radiography. It is defined as the ratio between the sagittal diameter of the vertebral body (BC) and the sagittal anteroposterior diameter of the posterior side of the sternum until the posterior side of the vertebral body (AC). The **L**ower **V**ertebral **I**ndex (**LVI**) is calculated at the xiphisternal junction [7, 10], whereas the **U**pper **V**ertebral **I**ndex (**UVI**) is calculated at the sternomanubrial junction [7].

Rebeis et al. [10] found that the LVI cut-off point for PE patients pre-operatively is within the means published by Derveaux et al., that is, 0.292 ± 0.067 (Fig. 7.2). Derveaux et al. [7] proposed three Chest-X-Ray indexes. The LVI (age dependent) was measured at the xiphisternal junction and calculated by BC/AC. The UVI (age independent) was measured at the sternomanubrial junction and calculated by EF/DF. The **Con**figuration **I**ndex (**ConI**) was the result of the ratio between DE/AB where DE and AB are the sagittal anteroposterior diameter of the back side of the sternum to the front side of the vertebral body, at the xiphisternal and sternomanubrial junctions, respectively. The ConI was particularly valuable in patients with complex PE, often with axial sternal rotation and/or scoliosis (Fig. 7.2). Mean pre-operative UVI was equal to 0.235 ± 0.045. Mean pre-operative ConI was equal to 1.175 ± 0.214. The results obtained regarding LVI were compatible

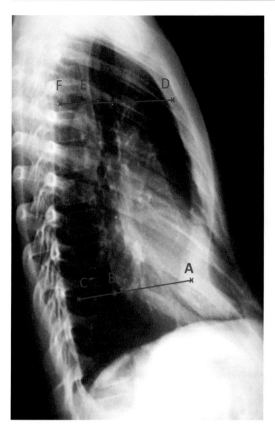

Fig. 7.2 Lateral Chest-X-Ray of a PE patient. Note Rebeis et al. and Derveaux et al. measurements to calculate the **Lower Vertebral Index** at the xiphisternal junction. *BC* = sagittal diameter of the vertebral body and *AC* = sagittal anteroposterior diameter of the back side of the sternum to the back side of the vertebral body. Derveaux et al. also measure the **Upper Vertebral Index** at the sternomanubrial junction. *EF* = sagittal diameter of the vertebral body and *DE* = sagittal anteroposterior diameter of the back side of the sternum to the back side of the vertebral body. The **Configuration Index** is the ratio between the sagittal anteroposterior diameter of the back side of the sternum to the front side of the vertebral body at the xiphisternal (*DE*) and sternomanubrial (*AB*) junctions

with those of Ohno et al. who expressed results as a percentage ratio. The pre-operative cut off point for LVI > 27 [16].

> **Lower Vertebral Index = BC/AC**
> **Upper Vertebral Index = EF/DF**
> **Configuration Index = DE/AB**

Frontosagittal Index

According to Ohno et al. the **F**ronto **S**agittal **I**ndex (**FSI**) is the percentage ratio between maximum internal transverse diameter (T) and minimum sagittal diameter of the chest, measured from the anterior surface of the vertebral body to the nearest point on the sternal body (D).

The authors concluded that the LVI decreased whereas the **FSI** increased significantly postoperatively (Fig. 7.3). They suspected that the abnormal post-operative indexes were the result of thin and flat chests, because of the short sagittal diameter of the thoracic cage, even though the sternum was adequately elevated and PE patients were satisfied with the cosmesis. The pre-operative cut off point for FSI < 29 [16].

> **Lower Vertebral Index = (B/A) × 100**
> **Fronto Sagittal Index = (D/T) × 100**

Welch Index

In 1958, Welch reported a technique for the correction of PE that emphasized total preservation of the perichondrial sheaths of the costal cartilage, preservation of the upper intercostal bundle, sternal osteotomy and anterior fixation of the sternum with silk sutures [17]. By the year 1988, Shamberger and Welch, had surgically corrected 704 PE patients with the same technique. Severity of the deformities was assessed on a scale 1–10 based on a series of measurements made from chest-x-rays (Fig. 7.4) [18]. According to the authors, surgical repair is recommended for PE patients beyond infancy with an inflexible deformity and a severity rating **Welch Index** (**WI**) of ≥5.

> **By calculating the:**
> 1. **Depression ratio (DR)** = D_1/D_2,
> 2. **Deformity Grade (DG)** = (1−DR) × 10 and the,

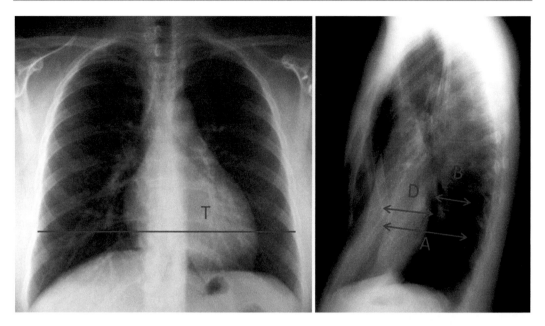

Fig. 7.3 PA and lateral Chest-X-Rays of a PE patient. **Lower Vertebral Index**: percentage ratio between minimum sagittal diameter of the chest measured from the posterior surface of the vertebral body to the nearest point on the sternal body (*A*) and the sagittal diameter of the vertebral body at the same level. (*B*) **Fronto Sagittal Index**: percentage ratio between maximum internal transverse diameter (*T*) and minimum sagittal diameter of the chest, measured from the anterior surface of the vertebral body to the nearest point on the sternal body (*D*)

3. **Cardiothoracic Ratio** = maximal horizontal cardiac diameter/maximal horizontal thoracic diameter (inner edge of ribs/edge of pleural) multiplied by 100. It is measured form a PA Chest-X-Ray. Normal values are <50 %.

The Welch Index is equal to:

– DG + 0.5 if Rib angle (Ø) > 25°

and/or

DG + 0.5 if the Cardiothoracic ratio >50 %

Haje Body Manubrial Index This sternal index has been proposed by Haje et al. It is obtained from a lateral chest X-ray. To calculate it, the length of the manubrium and body of the sternum are measured in centimeters. A ratio resultant of the division of the length of the ossified body (B) by the length of the ossified manubrium (M) is called the **B**ody **M**anubrium (**BM**) Index [2] (Fig. 7.5). It cannot be obtained when sternal segments are fused.

Body Manubrium Index = B/M

Haje Body Manubrium Xyphoid Index

This sternal index has also been proposed by Haje et al. It is obtained from a lateral Chest-X-Ray when ossification of the xyphoid process (X) is observed. A new ratio, representing the distance in centimeters from the top of the body to the bottom of the xyphoid process (BX) divided by the length of the manubrium (M), is obtained and called the **B**ody **M**anubrium **X**yphoid (**BXM**) Index (Fig. 7.5) [2].

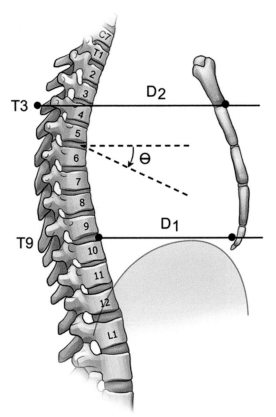

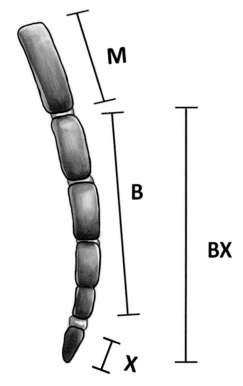

Fig. 7.5 Diagram of the measurements done on the lateral view of the sternum. (*M*) Manubrium length; (*B*) Body length; (*BX*) Body-Xyphoid distance. A lateral radiograph of a normal 11-year-old patient was used as a model

Fig. 7.4 Welch's method of grading severity of the deformity (Welch Index) uses the distance from the anterior surface of the spine at T-9 to the posterior surface of the sternum (*D-1*), over the distance from the spinous process of T-3 to the angle of Louis (*D-2*). Additional 0.5 is added if the rib angle (Ø) is greater than 25° or the cardiothoracic ratio is >50 %

> **Body Manubrium Xyphoid Index = BX/M**

The sternal body in controls is slightly more than twice the length of the manubrium. The cutoff point for the BM Index is 2.16 and for the BMX Index is 2.73. Lower BM values depict shorter sternal bodies.

The study originally aimed to determine the influence of sternal growth on the development of pectus deformities and correlate imaging studies with clinical aspects of different types of deformities. Although it was not Haje's main objective, when considering the BM and the BMX sternal indexes from a surgical point of view, these indexes might be useful to define surgical strategies as for example to predict the number of pectus bars needed for a Nuss procedure by correlating sternal length, age and thoracic elasticity.

Chest-X-ray Haller Index

The **H**aller **I**ndex (**HI**) will be explained in detail further in this chapter. It derives from dividing the greater transverse diameter (the horizontal distance of the inside of the ribcage) by the

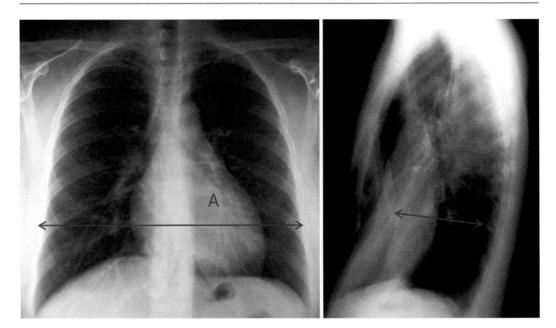

Fig. 7.6 **Chest-X-Ray Haller Index** measurement on two-view chest radiography. (*A*) The point of most posterior projection of the sternum is identified, and the distance between that segment and the anterior aspect of the corresponding vertebra is measured. (*B*) The lateral diameter is measured at the vertebral body level on the anteroposterior view

anteroposterior diameter (the shorter distance between the vertebrae and the sternum).

Poston et al. determined PE severity from Chest-X-Rays, instead of Chest CTs, to minimize radiation exposure of PE patients. Authors found a strong correlation between HIs calculated from Chest-X-Rays (Chest-X-Ray HIs) and those by Chest CT Scans. Both HIs demonstrated good inter-rater reliability. Nonetheless, even though the sensitivity of Chest-X-Rays in diagnosing severe PE (Chest CT HI≥3.2) resulted high, specificity was less convincing. But when using a cut-off point for Chest-X-Ray HIs of 3.75 or greater, combined specificity resulted quite high (0.96). They finally suggested using Chest CT Scans as a confirmatory test for Chest- X-Ray HIs between 3.2 and 3.75 [19].

According to Khanna et al. [20], Chest-X-Ray HI correlates strongly with Chest CT HI, has good inter-observer correlation, and a high diagnostic accuracy for pre-operative evaluation of PE. Authors suggest that a Chest CT is not required for pre-operative evaluation of PE, and a two-view Chest-X-Ray is sufficient enough for preoperative imaging of the defect.

Mueller et al. [21] measurements, calculated from preoperative Chest-X-Rays yielded HIs equivalent to those taken from Chest CT Scans. Authors postulated that the replacement of preoperative Chest CT by radiographies would reduce unnecessary exposure to radiation in children with asymptomatic PE. They believe this is particularly desirable because radiation exposure may have long-term side effects in growing children that range from long bone growth derangements to fatal malignancies. When in doubt, a Chest CT Scan could be indicated for the preoperative evaluation (Fig. 7.6).

Chest-X-Ray Haller Index = A/B

Chest Scan Indexes

Haje Width Length Index

This index was proposed by Haje et al. from coronal CT Scans, traced out on a schematic representation of the anterior chest wall. The **W**idth **L**ength **I**ndex (**WLI**) is calculated by dividing

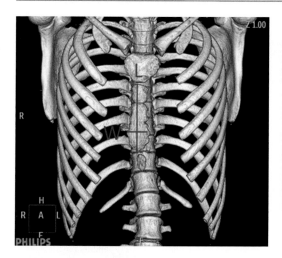

Fig. 7.7 Lines *W* (widest length of the ossified sternal body) and *L* (longest length of the ossified sternal body), are used for the study of the WL index in coronal CT Scans. The **Width Length Index** is calculated by the division of W by L

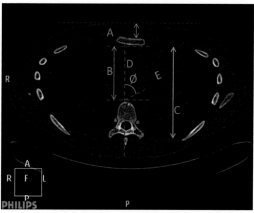

Fig. 7.8 Chest CT Scan showing measurements to calculate the depth of sternal depression (*A*), **Sternal Depression Index** (*C/B*), and cardiac rotation angle (*Ø*). *D*=sagittal line from anterior border of the vertebral body and line from anterior border of vertebral body (*E*)

the maximum width of the ossified sternal body by its length (Fig. 7.7). This implies higher WLI indexes for wide sternal bodies, with possible connotations for the prognosis and treatment of different types of pectus deformities [1]. The mean WLI Index for controls is 0.420. The mean WLI Index for PE patients is >0.446.

$$\text{Width Length Index} = W/L$$

Sternal Depression Index

The Sternal Depression Index (**SDI**) is the ratio between the maximal internal sagittal diameter of the left side of the chest (C) and the minimal distance between the anterior surface of the vertebral column and the posterior border of the deepest portion of the sternum (B).

The vertical distance between the higher and lowest point of the anterior chest wall (A) is a measure of the sternal depression.

Chu et al. [30] reported that the average depth of depression of the sternum (A) was 21±7 mm whereas the SDI was 2.7±1.4. When the SDI was arbitrarily used to classify the severity of sternal deformity, mild sternal deformity was associated to a SDI<2.4; moderate sternal deformity was

associated to a SDI between 2.4 and 2.9; and severe sternal deformity was associated to a SDI index >2.9 (Fig. 7.8). As the depression index increased, the cardiac rotation angle (Ø) increased with a correlation coefficient of 0.75.

Haller Index

The Haller Index (**HI**), described in 1987 by Dr. Haller J, Dr. Kramer and Dr. Lietman, is a mathematical relationship, usually measured by chest CT scans [22]. As aforementioned, HI derives from dividing the transverse diameter (the widest horizontal distance of the inside of the ribcage) [T] by the anteroposterior diameter (the shorter distance between the vertebrae and the sternum) [A] (Fig. 7.9) [23].

$$\text{Haller Index} = T/A$$

Despite several issues that will be discussed further, the HI remains a useful tool in judgment of operative indication. The cut-off point for PE patients is >3.25 [22].

The HI has been chosen as the gold standard for the majority of chest wall malformation experts. Presumably because it is easy to measure, and because surgeons and radiologists are

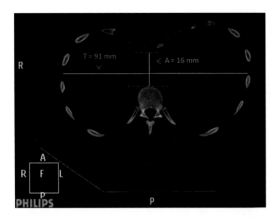

Fig. 7.9 CT axial image: Calculation of the *Haller Index* = 91 mm/16 mm = 5.68. The sternum is so severely depressed that it is 1.6 cm from the anterior portion of the vertebra

Table 7.2 Limitations of the Haller Index

Problems with the Haller Index (thoroughly documented in the literature)	
Fairness (for patients and surgeons)	3.25 cut-off point for surgical indication is no longer a good discriminator between PE patients and controls [4, 20, 28, 41]
	Bares no conclusive relationship with the aesthetic complaints observed [24, 41]
	Variation with thoracic shape [2, 5, 41]
	Variation with age and gender [4, 5]
	Variation with inspiration/expiration [24]
	Depends on chest width which results in overlapping between controls and PE patients [26]
Practicity	Does not consider asymmetry [27–29, 41–44]
	Does not consider cardiac compression [29, 31, 38]

used to calculate and interpret it. Moreover, it has a high inter-observational reliability as demonstrated by Lawson et al. [41] Nonetheless, it is thoroughly documented that the HI has several limitations (Table 7.2).

To start with, there is no convincing evidence regarding it provides accurate information to guide surgical correction of PE. Its cut-off point is quite variable among authors. Daunt et al. [4] for instance proposed an upper limit of 2.7, Khanna et al. [20] of 3.2, Kilda et al. [43] of 3.1 whereas most chest wall malformation experts adopt a cut-off point equal or greater than 3.25. In spite of this, as Lawson et al. [41] published, there is a considerable variability among medical practitioners in determining the HI depending on how the images are chosen and how measurements are taken from the chosen images. Secondly, the HI might be unreliable since it varies with age, gender [4, 5], thoracic shape [2, 5], and whether it is done in inspiration or expiration [30]. Thirdly HI is unpractical for surgical – decision making as it does not consider asymmetry [24], percentage of sternal and costal depression [24], cardiac compression or cardiac asymmetry [41, 44]. Also results from controls and PE patients overlap between each other [26]. While width serves as a surrogate for comparing dimensions of the chest, it does not depict the position of the sternum relative to the anterior ribcage. A wide chest increases HI whereas a narrow chest decreases HI regardless of the severity of the

PE [24]. HI bares no conclusive relationship with the aesthetic complaints observed. For instance, the patient in (Fig. 7.10) clearly has a PE. But when calculating his HI it is equal to 3.24. St. Peter et al. proposed the Correction Index (CI), a novel thoracic index, which is independent of chest width and assesses the percentage of chest depth [26]. The CI will be described ahead in this chapter.

Modified Haller Indexes

The Modified Haller Indexes result from changes made to the HI.

Haller Index in Expiration

Chest wall diameters vary with breathing and these variations may modify the **H**aller **I**ndex in **Ex**piration (**HI-Ex**) values and surgical indications [25]. Albertal et al. found that the antero-posterior diameter values vary from end-inspiration to end-expiration, and correspond to significant changes (29.6 %) in HI values (Fig. 7.11) [24]. Their study showed that HI was more severe at end-expiration than at end-inspiration, leading to an increase in surgical candidacy.

Haller Index for Carinatum

The **H**aller **I**ndex for **C**arinatum (**HI-Car**) is a kind of "reverse" HI described by Poncet et al. [40]

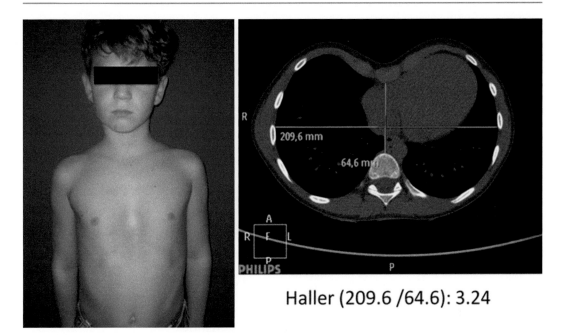

Haller (209.6 /64.6): 3.24

Fig. 7.10 (*Left*) Patient consulting for PE. (*Right*) Chest CT Scan revealing a Haller Index = 3.24. According to the cut-off point of HI, the patient does not have PE

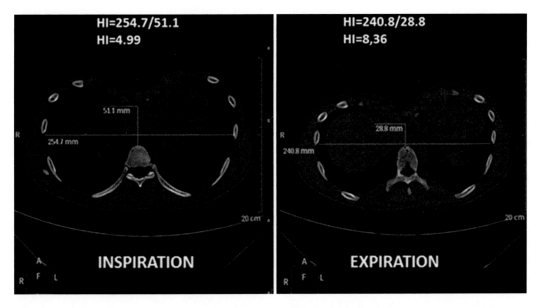

Fig. 7.11 Chest CT Scan of a 16-year-old PE patient. Axial CT images of the same patient are observed at full inspiration and full expiration. Demonstration of measurements performed to assess PE. A significant reduction in the anteroposterior diameter of the chest at full expiration can be noted, while minimal change is observed in the transverse diameter

Authors calculated severity indexes of the deformities from Chest CT scans and from the outline of torso cross sections (i.e., from skin to skin measurements) obtained from optical images. To assess the severity of carinatum defects, the HI-Car (*d*Lat/*d*AP) and a modified pectus index (**moHI-Car**) –

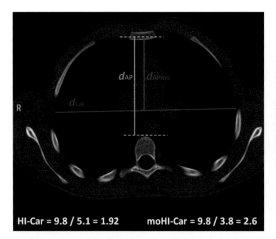

HI-Car = 9.8 / 5.1 = 1.92   moHI-Car = 9.8 / 3.8 = 2.6

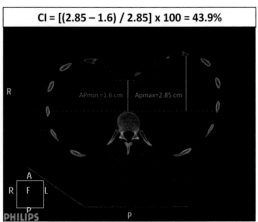

CI = [(2.85 – 1.6) / 2.85] x 100 = 43.9%

Fig. 7.12 Haller Index for Pectus Carinatum: the widest transverse diameter [*dLAT*] is divided by the highest antero-posterior distance [*dAP*]. **Chest CT Haller Index adapted for pectus carinatum**: the widest transverse diameter [*dLAT*] divided by the distance from the central chord to the under surface of the maximal protrusion [*dAPmo*]

Fig. 7.13 Calculation of the **Correction Index**. In this case it is almost 44 % indicating the patient has a moderate to severe PE

which calculates the ratio between the central chord to the under surface of the maximal protrusion (**dAPmo**) by the widest transverse diameter (**dLat**) (Fig. 7.12) – were measured. Values of HI-Car ranged from 1.19 to 2.2 (mean=1.66). Values of Chest CT moHI-Car ranged from 2.27 to 3.1 (mean=2.5). Regression analyses were performed to compare results from both Chest-CT HI-Car and Chest-CT moHI-Car with results from cross- sections of HI -Car and moHI-car obtained from optical images. Optical measures of cross-sectional deformities correlated well with HI-Car (r^2=0.94) and even better with those of moHI-Car (r^2=0.96). According to the authors, adaptation of the Haller Index for pectus carinatum deformity evaluation was effective, and consistent with the torso surface deformity measures.

> **Haller Index for Carinatum**=*d*Lat/*d*AP
> **Modified Haller Index for Carinatum**= *d*Lat/*d*APmo

Correction Index

The Correction Index (**CI**) was described by St. Peter et al. [26] who observed that HI is dependent on width and does not assess the depth of the defect correctly. In their study by utilizing larger cohorts with age-defined groups for controls they concluded that using a height to width ratio of 3.25 as a discriminator to define potential candidates for PE repair could no longer be held true.

Thereby the authors proposed a novel index calculated from chest CT at end-inspiration [26].

A horizontal line is drawn across the anterior spine. Then the CI measures the minimum distance between the posterior sternum and the anterior spine (narrowest point) [AP min], plus the maximum distance between the anterior spine and the anterior portion of the chest (widest point) [AP max]. The difference between those values (widest minus narrowest point), in other words, the amount of defect, is divided by the widest point (Fig. 7.13) and finally multiplied by 100 thus giving the percentage of PE depth the patient is missing. Conversely, it represents the percentage of chest depth to be corrected by bar placement.

Using the CI, a normal distribution is created more clearly for both controls and PE patients with no overlap between them. The gap is in fact large enough to enable a high degree of confidence in defining PE. The key to CI success is that it is blind to chest width and that it defines the distance of the sternum from the goal position.

> **Correction Index = [(AP max–AP min)/ AP max] × 100**

The cut-off point of CI is set at 10 % to differentiate controls from PE patients without overlapping. St. Peter et al. [26] statistically demonstrated that a CI > 10 % means that more than 10 % of the chest depth between the anterior chest and the anterior spine is centrally depressed which is by definition PE. With this novel index, the possibility of a high index and no defect or a deep defect with a low index is removed.

Poston et al. [19] validated the findings of St. Peter et al. [26], using the same formula but calculating the CI differently. They recommend a CI of 28 % or greater when correlating statistically with the well known Haller Index cut-off value of 3.25 (which unfortunately has never been validated). These authors also observed that although the HI correlates well with the CI in PE patients with symmetric chest wall deformities, it is quite discrepant in asymmetric cases.

Deformity Indexes

According to Lawson et al. [41] deformity indexes are needed because the HI alone may be inadequate to quantify postoperative changes in the shape of the chest. Individual PE patients may also have chest characteristics that impact the success of repair, many of which would be unlikely to be measured solely by the HI.

They thereby designed a digitizer protocol used by radiologists, which included detailed instructions on how to select the appropriate 5 images to calculate pectus defect severity. Once the measurements were made, the HI and

Asymmetry Index (AI) were calculated for each slice as T/A and R/L × 100, respectively. A patient's overall HI was defined as the largest of the 5 images calculated. Both radiologists disagreed with the 3.2 threshold used as the cut-off point for eligibility for surgery by insurance companies and numerous surgeons. The AI was defined as the farthest from 100 of the 5 images' calculated value. For this reliability study, the indexes were compared between digitizer measurements and between radiologists for each slice selected. The radiologists had almost perfect agreement on the selection of the slices to be used for the HI and AI. They noted the use of the cross-sectional area is less likely to be impacted by the shape of the chest than any currently used index. The digitizer protocol alleviated potential biases and inconsistencies in data being collected from multiple centers with competing surgical treatments. Although it is more extensive than just determining a single HI or AI as a rough gauge of severity or deformity, it provides a tool for assessing both the need for surgery and the outcome of repair in any future quality monitoring program or to readily study any potential future modifications of the surgical technique (Fig. 7.14) [41].

> **Asymmetry Index = (R/L) × 100**
> Interpretation:
> When AI = 100; R = L; Symmetric PE
> When AI > 100; R > L; Right Asymmetric PE
> When AI < 100: R < L; Left Asymmetric PE
> This Asymmetry Index is expressed as a percentage ratio

Other surgeons preferred deformity indexes such as the **V**ertebral **I**ndex (**VI**) and the **F**ronto **S**agittal **I**ndex (**FSI**) to evaluate the degree of chest wall deformation changes after surgery, using pre- and postoperative radiological examination data.

Kilda et al., for example, concluded that when preparing a PE patient for surgery, it is important

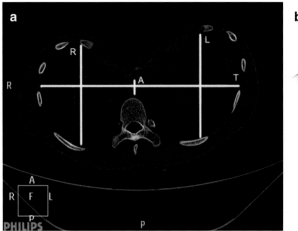 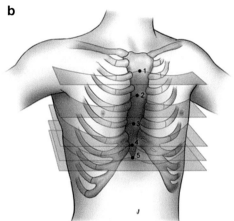

Fig. 7.14 (a) Axial CT Scan of a patient with PE. Calculation of the Haller Index and Asymmetry Index. Ref: [T] transversal chest dimension; [R and L] sagittal right and left chest size dimensions; [A] sternovertebral distance. (b) 5-position protocol for intrathoracic measurement of Haller Index and Asymmetry Index at each cut level. Position 1: the level of the sternomanubrial junction (anterior second rib ends); Position 5: the level of the tip of the xiphoid; Position 4: the level of the end of the body of the sternum; Positions 2 and 3: divide the distance between positions 1 and 4 by 3. Position 2 is one third of the way between positions 1 and 4, and position 3 is two thirds of the way between positions 1 and 4 (calculated by the digitizer technician)

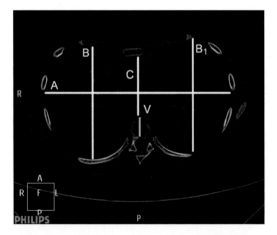

Fig. 7.15 Axial CT scan showing value assessments. [A] transversal chest dimension. [B and B_1] sagittal right and left chest size dimensions. [C] sternovertebral distance. [V] vertebral body length

Vertebral Index $= [\text{V}/(\text{V}+\text{C})] \times 100$
Frontosagittal Index $= (\text{C}/\text{A}) \times 100$

Masaoka et al. calculated the steepness index, excavatum volume index and asymmetry index to evaluate the impact of surgical repair on PE patients (Fig. 7.16) [27]. Pre- and postoperative means were estimated for each index but no information about cut-off points was given though.

All measurements improved postoperatively.

Steepness Index $= \text{D}/\text{W}$
Excavation Volume Index $= \text{O} \times \text{W}/ (\text{IA} \times \text{IB}) + (\text{rA} \times \text{rB})$
Asymmetry Index $= \text{IA} \times \text{IB}/\text{rA} \times \text{rB}$

to perform a chest CT scan and give an overall evaluation of the chest shape and deformation degree considering the following cut-off points: VI > 26, FSI < 33 and HI > 3.1 They also concluded the dynamics of deformation is better depicted by means of VI rather than HI (Fig. 7.15) [43, 44].

Lee et al. [28] retrospectively analyzed pre- and postoperative Chest CTs of more than 300 PE patients to obtain new CT indexes: **D**epression

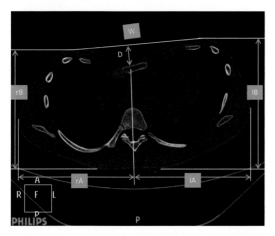

Fig. 7.16 Masaoka et al.'s measurements for deformity indexes *W* distance between the prominent points of the anterior chest wall on both sides, *D* length of the perpendicular line between the center of the anterior table of the sternum and the line showing combination of both prominent points, *rA* length between the right lateral thoracic wall and the vertical line from the center of sternum, *rB* distance between the prominent point of right anterior thoracic wall and the touch line of right back, *IA* length between the left lateral thoracic wall and the vertical line from the center of the sternum, *IB* distance between the prominent point of left anterior thoracic wall and the touch line of left back

Index (**DI**), **A**symmetry Index (**AI**), **E**ccentricity Index and Unbalance Index. These were useful in precise understanding of the degrees of depression and asymmetries as well as in comparing morphological changes before and after operative repair of the defect (Fig. 7.17). Evaluation of the AI revealed that treating PE patients with the Nuss technique enabled symmetrical correction of asymmetric PE. Lee et al. postulated that with the modified techniques tailored to each specific type of asymmetry, indications of the Nuss procedure could be expanded essentially to all morphological kinds of PE.

The four thoracic indexes decreased after surgery. When comparing preoperative values of symmetric and asymmetric PE AI values were different (1.036 ± 0.042 vs. 1.107 ± 0.080, $p < 0.01$), but postoperatively the difference became not significant (1.019 ± 0.022 vs. 1.024 ± 0.028, $p = 0.08$), which means asymmetric types are corrected to a symmetric configuration after surgery [28].

Cartoski et al. [6] calculated the HI by T/A, **A**symmetry Index (**AI**) by R/L × 100, and Chest

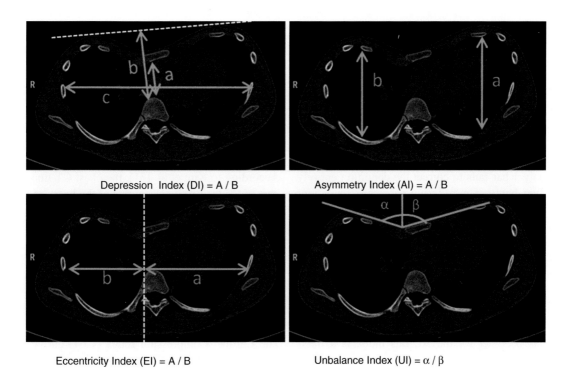

Depression Index (DI) = A / B

Asymmetry Index (AI) = A / B

Eccentricity Index (EI) = A / B

Unbalance Index (UI) = α / β

Fig. 7.17 Deformity indexes displaying degrees of Depression, Asymmetry, Eccentricity, and Unbalance

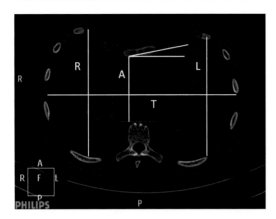

Fig. 7.18 Deformity indexes displaying severity of the Depression, Asymmetry, Chest shape and Torsion angle

Shape Index by T/R. Sternal torsion angle is marked and represents the degree of torsion or tilt to the right (most common) or left (unfrequent). All measurements were measured at maximum distances except for A, which was measured as the minimum distance between the anterior surface of the vertebral column and the deepest portion of the sternum (Fig. 7.18).

Asymmetry Index = R/L × 100
Chest Shape Index = T/R

The authors point out that a long PE has surgical relevance relating to choices made during the corrective procedure. The Nuss procedure may require 2 bars instead of 1 if the patient has a depression affecting the chest that the addition of only 1 bar fails to correct the condition entirely. Two bars are not always necessary for a long depression as some patients, especially younger children, have greater flexibility in their thoracic cavity and experience a good correction with a single bar.

Chest CT scans allow greater perception of asymmetry inside the thoracic cavity in comparison with the external clinical perception. Although no cut-off point for surgical eligibility has been set for the AI, this index is a likely

predictor of surgical outcome. Since it is a ratio of two sides of the PE depression values away from 100 are merely a reflection of whether the right or the left side of the depression is deeper.

Sternal torsion measured at an angle >30° is considered severe, whereas mild torsion is applied to any angle <30°. Sternal torsion to the right often appears with asymmetry to the right and the other way around in general. A sternal torsion to the left changes the surgical strategy to avoid injuring the heart. A severely twisted sternum upon correction does not always completely flatten and can leave a slight protuberance in the appearance of the chest.

Kim et al. [29] believe conventional indexes that define the severity of PE have several limitations, e.g. they are manually calculated and cannot supply information about asymmetry. The authors developed four automatized indexes that can represent both the depression and the asymmetry of the chest-wall by CT Scan. Three indexes, including **E**ccentricity **I**ndex (**EI**), **F**latness **I**ndex (**FI**), and **C**ircularity **I**ndex (**CI**), were suggested to represent the depression of the chest-wall, and one index, **R**otation **I**ndex (**RI**), to represent the asymmetry of the chest-wall. The suggested indexes showed clear trends of change with the severity of chest-wall deformation in regards to both the depression and the asymmetry. Results of statistical analysis showed high correlation between the new indexes and HI, showing possibility of replacing HI.

Cardiac Compression and Cardiac Asymmetry Index

According to Kim et al. [31], the chest CT findings of PE include displacement of the heart into the left hemithorax with mild clockwise rotation and a pancake-like appearance of the heart with an increase of the frontal silhouette to the left. The possible mechanisms that produce circulatory problems include: (1) decreased inflow due to cardiac rotation and twisting of the great veins; (2) cardiac compression; (3) impaired diastolic expansion; and (4) decreased respiratory effort. The **C**ardiac **C**ompression **I**ndex (**CCI**) derives from the H/M ratio and the **C**ardiac **A**symmetry Index (**CAI**) derives from the P/M ratio (Fig. 7.19).

Modified Cardiac Compression Index

Albertal et al. [24] calculated the cardiac compression index (CCI) from chest CT by dividing the cardiac transverse diameter by the cardiac antero-posterior diameter. CCI increased significantly during end-expiration, primarily driven by an increase on the cardiac transverse diameter.

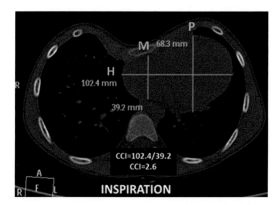

Fig. 7.19 Calculation of the Cardiac Compression Index (*CCI*) and the Cardiac Asymmetry Index (CAI) from a Chest CT at end-inspiration. CCI=102.4/39.2=2.6 (Cut-off point: 1.82); CAI=68.3/39.2=1.74 (Cut-off point 1.15)

Surgical indication was found in 71 % and 91 % (20 % difference) of patients during end-inspiration and end-expiration, respectively ($p < 0.05$) (Fig. 7.20). Authors therefore recommend performing the CT at end-expiration.

MRI Indexes

These include all the aforementioned indexes and cardiac indexes for delineating the anatomical and physiological components of PE as well as measuring the results of treatment [32]. As already said, the diagnoses of PE is clinical. Nonetheless the quantitative measurement of the deformity has been evaluated by means of radiographies and CTs. Recent reports in the literature have recognized the problem of radiation and some authors commenced using MRI to diagnose and assess the severity of the pectus deformity [33–35]. Future directions could eventually include the routine acquisition of inspiratory and expiratory MRI sequences. Research has shown that this may provide more physiological information; in expiration, the deformity may worsen [36]. Furthermore, cine MRI has demonstrated to be capable of evaluating both chest morphology and chest wall kinetics, and may well add important diagnostic information [45].

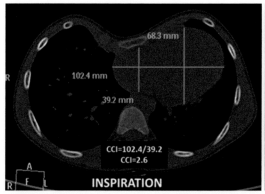

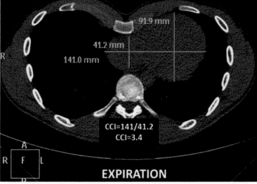

Fig. 7.20 Axial images of the heart at full inspiration and full expiration. Measurements performed to assess cardiac compression are shown. There is a significant increase in the cardiac transverse diameter at full expiration and no

valuable modifications in the cardiac anteroposterior diameter. Notice the maximal cardiac anteroposterior diameter revealed a sizeable increase of 5.1 % at full expiration whereas the maximal cardiac transverse diameter, 37.7 %

Survey

Because of the large number of thoracic indexes reported worldwide and the diverse variety of diagnostic tools available today, there is no consensus on which is the best thoracic index to diagnose, assess severity, define strategies within treatment, and quantify postoperative thoracic shape changes. For this reason, a selected group of international chest wall malformations experts were consulted by means of a web-based survey. The main objective was to start classifying thoracic indexes and to establish a unifying criterion.

The entire project was designed, implemented and analyzed by Drs. Martinez-Ferro and Park, and supervised by the Chest Wall International Group (CWIG) president, Dr. H. Pilegaard. The web-based survey was performed using the Survey Monkey™ (Palo Alto, CA, USA) website. It consisted of 10 multiple choice questions about the preoperative and intraoperative management of PE patients, focusing on the current use of the most commonly used thoracic indexes for surgical planning. In general, more than one answer could be selected per question. The survey was confidential and anonymous (Table 7.3).

Table 7.3 Ten multiple-choice questionnaire. Web-based survey

(Q1) Which preoperative studies do you use in ALL (100 %) your patients with pectus excavatum?
Chest X-ray
Chest CT
3D Chest CT
MRI
Cardiac MRI
Cardiac US
Echo stress
Cardiopulmonary test
Exercise stress test
24-h Holter monitoring
Pulmonary function test
Plethismography
Thoracic spine X-ray
Nickel allergy test and/or other metal allergy tests
Other (describe)
(Q2) In your opinion, thoracic indexes for treatment decision-making are?
Essential
Very useful
Barely needed
Useless
(Q3) If a, b or c, why do you use them?
Because Insurance Companies/Health System request them
Because they help you to identify the severity of the deformity
Because they may change the surgical technique and/or approach
Because they help you describe the problem to the patient
I don't use them at all

(Q4) Which Indexes do you routinely use in your practice?
Haller Index
Modified Haller Index
Correction Index
Welch Index (X-ray)
Asymmetry Index
Cross-sectional chest area
Depression Index
Eccentricity Index
Flatness Index
Circularity Index
Unbalance Index
CT-derived Cardiac Compression Index
CT-derived Correction Index (Kansas)
Anthropometric Index
Vertebral Index
Frontosagittal Index
Other (describe)
(Q5) The Haller Index is:
Essential
Very useful
Useful
Useless
(Q6) In your opinion, a 3.25 Haller index as cut-off value between surgical and non-surgical patients is:
Correct
Incorrect
(Q7) You order a Haller Index
In inspiration
In expiration
I do not specify it in my order

Table 7.3 (continued)

(Q8) If you had to choose only one Index to use, which one would you prefer?
Haller Index
Modified Haller Index
Correction Index
Welch Index (X-ray)
Asymmetry Index
Cross-sectional chest area
Depression Index
Eccentricity Index
Flatness Index
Circularity Index
Unbalance Index
CT-derived Cardiac Compression Index
CT-derived Correction Index (Kansas)
Anthropometric Index
Vertebral Index
Frontosagittal Index
Other (describe)
(Q9) Which is your preferred technique for the correction of pectus excavatum?
Resective surgery (Ravitch and modifications)
Nuss Technique (and modifications)
Bardaji Ventura Technique
Other (specify)
(Q10) If you selected the "Nuss Technique", would you consider important to have a way of predicting in advance how many bars will the patient need?
Yes
No

The invitation, together with 3 reminders, were sent to chest wall malformation experts between March and April 2014. After the 2 months prospective data collection period, responses were downloaded to a Microsoft Excel™ file (Redmond, WA, USA) for descriptive analyses of answers. Duplicate responses corresponding to the same author were removed by deleting the less complete response.

Results

Of the 334 surveyed chest wall malformation experts, 92 answered the questions and a mean of 86, range: 92–74 (25.74 %) participated in the project. Sixty-one percent were males.

In accordance with **Question 1 (Q1)**, for preoperative evaluation, 58.7 % of responders tend to indicate a Chest CT Scan whereas 50.2 %, order a Chest X-Ray and/or an Echocardiography. A 3D Chest CT Scan is opted by 22.8 % of the PE experts, and a Thoracic Spine – X – Ray, by only 7.6 % of them. Nobody will indicate a cardiac MRI or a Plethismography. Moreover, while 50 % of the surgeons always request a pulmonary function test, those exams involving exercise (as treadmill exercise, stress-echo US or cardiopulmonar tests) are seemingly to be ordered by only a 12 % (Fig. 7.21).

Question 2 (Q2) is about the value of thoracic indexes for treatment decision-making, 14.3 % of chest wall malformation experts reported they are essential; 45 %, very useful; 35.1 % barely needed and 5.6 % useless (Fig. 7.22).

The reason for using thoracic indexes is detailed in the answers to **Question 3 (Q3)**.

Forty-four of those who do not consider thoracic indexes useless (72.1 %), employ them because they help to better identify the severity of the deformity and 30 (49.2 %), because thoracic indexes help to describe the problem to the patient. Insurance Companies/Health Systems are a less significant reason, and only 13.51 % of the surgeons will use thoracic indexes to change their surgical technique and/or approach (Fig. 7.23).

According to **Question 4 (Q4)**, 89.78 % of responders prefer to employ in their routine practice either the Haller Index (79.55 %) or a modified Haller Index (10.23 %) (Fig. 7.24).

In **Question 5 (Q5)** 86.36 % of the surgeons consider the Haller Index: Essential, Useful and Very Useful (Fig. 7.25).

Surprisingly more than half of the experts (56.32 %) consider a cut-off value of 3.25 incorrect, **Question 6 (Q6)**, (Fig. 7.26). This seems to be a contradiction when considering that the analysis of Q4 and Q5 reveal that almost 90 % responders indicate a Haller Index routinely, and 86.36 % believe it is essential, useful and very useful.

Results of Q6 are also in conflict with those revealed in **Question 8 (Q8)**, as almost 70 % of responders state that they prefer the Haller Index

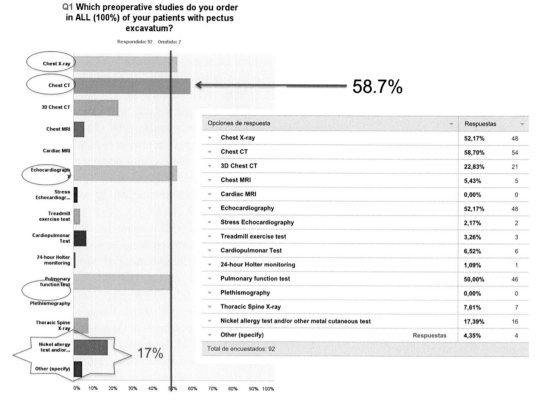

Q1 Which preoperative studies do you order in ALL (100%) of your patients with pectus excavatum?

Respondido: 92   Omitido: 2

Opciones de respuesta	Respuestas	
Chest X-ray	52,17%	48
Chest CT	58,70%	54
3D Chest CT	22,83%	21
Chest MRI	5,43%	5
Cardiac MRI	0,00%	0
Echocardiography	52,17%	48
Stress Echocardiography	2,17%	2
Treadmill exercise test	3,26%	3
Cardiopulmonar Test	6,52%	6
24-hour Holter monitoring	1,09%	1
Pulmonary function test	50,00%	46
Plethismography	0,00%	0
Thoracic Spine X-ray	7,61%	7
Nickel allergy test and/or other metal cutaneous test	17,39%	16
Other (specify) Respuestas	4,35%	4
Total de encuestados: 92		

Fig. 7.21 Question 1 results

Fig. 7.22 Question 2 results

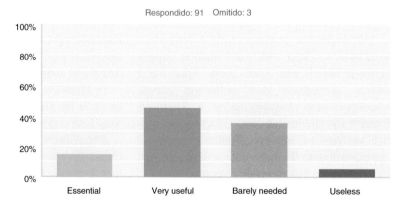

Q2 In your opinion for treatment decision-making, Thoracic Indexes are:

Respondido: 91   Omitido: 3

or a modified Haller Index if they had to choose only one single index (Fig. 7.27).

When asking if the Haller Index should be ordered in Inspiration or Expiration in Question 7 (**Q7**), 65.48 % reported it is irrelevant, whereas 19.05 % and 15.48 % said they request it during expiration and inspiration, respectively (Fig. 7.28).

Fig. 7.23 Question 3 results

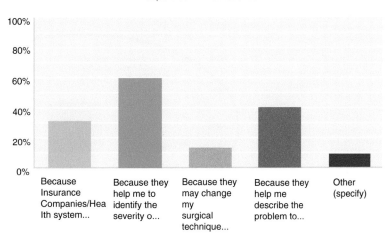

Q3 If not useless, why do you use Thoracic Indexes?

Respondido: 74   Omitido: 20

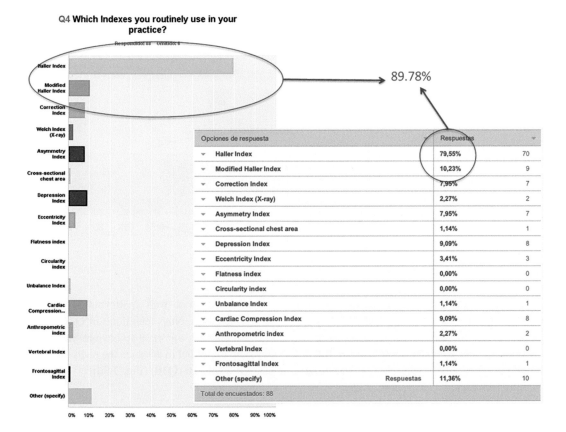

Fig. 7.24 Question 4 results

Fig. 7.25 Question 5 results

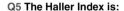

Q5 The Haller Index is:

Respondido: 88   Omitido: 6

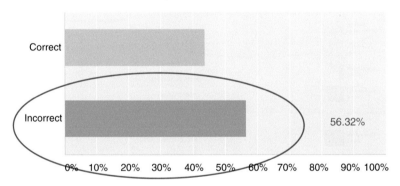

86.36%

100%

80%

60%

40%

20%

0%

Essential   Very useful   Useful   Useless

Fig. 7.26 Question 6 results

Q6 In your opinion, a 3.25 Haller index as cut-off value between surgical and non-surgical patients is:

Respondido: 87   Omitido: 7

Correct

Incorrect

56.32%

0% 10% 20% 30% 40% 50% 60% 70% 80% 90% 100%

Question **9** (**Q9**) is about the preferred surgical technique for the correction of PE. Most surgeons (89.53 %) advocate PE repair with the Nuss technique, whereas a few use the Ravitch procedure (3.49 %) or its variants, or the Bardaji – Ventura technique (1.16 %) (Fig. 7.29).

For those chest wall malformation experts who selected the Nuss technique in Question 9, 75.9 % consider important to have an index that may help to predict in advance the need for 1 or 2 bars. Question **10** (**Q10**) (Fig. 7.30).

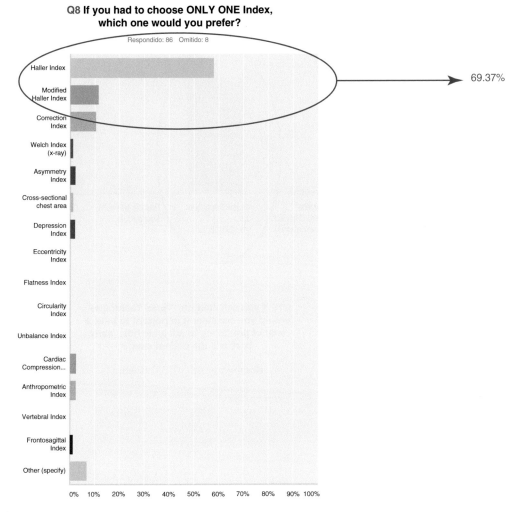

Fig. 7.27 Question 8 results

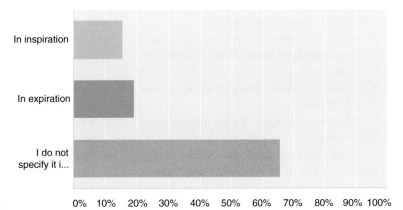

Fig. 7.28 Question 7 results

Fig. 7.29 Question 9 results

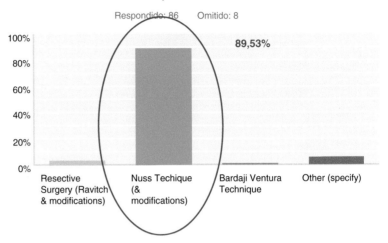

Q9 Which is your preferred technique for the correction of pectus excavatum?

Fig. 7.30 Question 10 results

Q10 If you selected the "Nuss Technique", would you consider it important to have a way of predicting in advance how many bars will the patient need?

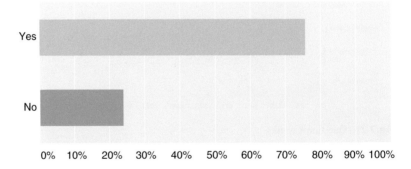

Conclusions

The survey revealed the need to:

- establish an order and propose a classification for the large variety of thoracic indexes in existence,
- replace the Haller Index and find a new gold standard,
- validate all indexes before putting them into practice

After analyzing them one by one in this chapter, it has to be concluded that there is currently no thoracic index without limitations. Perhaps the perfect index will be a mathematical combination of several different indexes. Perhaps it will be a single index still to be discovered. In any case, the index must be a diagnostic and assessment tool that will enable to:

1. Establish the difference between PE patients and controls without overlapping.
2. Evaluate the severity of the deformity without biases.
3. Quantify the cardiopulmonary impact of the deformity without biases
4. Help to define therapeutical strategies
5. Quantify improvements after surgical repair or after non-operative treatment.

Most probably this effort could only be achieved by an international "task-force" composed by experts working in centers with vast experience in treating thoracic wall deformities. In this case, there is room for a society such as the Chest Wall International Group that gather many of such experts and centers. It may take many years to find a universal, validated thoracic index, but the labor will be worthwhile.

References

1. Haje SA, Haje Dde P, Silva Neto M, e Cassia Gde S, Batista RC, de Oliveira GR, Mundim TL. Pectus deformities: tomographic analysis and clinical correlation. Skeletal Radiol. 2010;39(8):773–82.
2. Haje SA, Harcke HT, Bowen JR. Growth disturbance of the sternum and pectus deformities: imaging studies and clinical correlation. Pediatr Radiol. 1999;29(5):334–41.
3. Haje SA, Haje Dde P. Abordagem ortopédica das deformidades pectus: 32 anos de estudos. Rev Bras Ortop. 2009;44(3):191–8.
4. Daunt SW, Cohen JH, Miller SF. Age-related normal ranges for the Haller index in children. Pediatr Radiol. 2004;34(4):326–30.
5. Rebeis EB, Campos JR, Moreira LF, Pastorino AC, Pêgo-Fernandes PM, Jatene FB. Variation of the Anthropometric Index for pectus excavatum relative to age, race, and sex. Clinics (Sao Paulo). 2013; 68(9):1215–9.
6. Cartoski MJ, Nuss D, Goretsky MJ, Proud VK, Croitoru DP, Gustin T, Mitchell K, Vasser E, Kelly Jr RE. Classification of the dysmorphology of pectus excavatum. J Pediatr Surg. 2006;41(9):1573–81.
7. Derveaux L, Clarysse I, Ivanoff I, Demedts M. Preoperative and postoperative abnormalities in chest x-ray indices and in lung function in pectus deformities. Chest. 1989;95(4):850–6.
8. Malek MH, Berger DE, Housh TJ, Marelich WD, Coburn JW, Beck TW. Cardiovascular function following surgical repair of pectus excavatum: a meta-analysis. Chest. 2006;130(2):506–16. Review.
9. Maagaard M, Tang M, Ringgaard S, Nielsen HH, Frøkiær J, Haubuf M, Pilegaard HK, Hjortdal VE. Normalized cardiopulmonary exercise function in patients with pectus excavatum three years after operation. Ann Thorac Surg. 2013;96(1):272–8.
10. Rebeis EB, Campos JR, Fernandez A, Moreira LF, Jatene FB. Anthropometric index for pectus excavatum. Clinics (Sao Paulo). 2007;62(5):599–606.
11. Knutson U. Measurement of thoracic deformities. A new technique giving objective and reproducible results. Scand J Thorac Cardiovasc Surg. 1967; 1(1):76–9.
12. Horst M, Albrecht D, Drerup B. Objective determination of the shape of the anterior chest wall using moiré topography. Method and development of dimension-free indices for the evaluation of funnel chest. Z Orthop Ihre Grenzgeb. 1985;123(3):357–64. German.
13. Backer OG, Brunner S, Larsen V. The surgical treatment of funnel chest. Initial and follow-up results. Acta Chir Scand. 1961;121:253–61.
14. Backer OG, Brunner S, Larsen V. Radiologic evaluation of funnel chest. Acta Radiol. 1961;55:249–56.
15. Hümmer HP, Willital GH. Morphologic findings of chest deformities in children corresponding to the Willital-Hümmer classification. J Pediatr Surg. 1984;19(5):562–6.
16. Ohno K, Nakahira M, Takeuchi S, Shiokawa C, Moriuchi T, Harumoto K, Nakaoka T, Ueda M, Yoshida T, Tsujimoto K, Kinoshita H. Indications for surgical treatment of funnel chest by chest radiograph. Pediatr Surg Int. 2001;17(8):591–5.
17. Welch KJ. Satisfactory surgical correction of pectus excavatum deformity in childhood; a limited opportunity. J Thorac Surg. 1958;36(5):697–713.
18. Shamberger RC, Welch KJ. Surgical repair of pectus excavatum. J Pediatr Surg. 1988;23(7):615–22.
19. Poston PM, Patel SS, Rajput M, Rossi NO, Davis JE, Turek JW. Defining the role of chest radiography in determining candidacy for pectus excavatum repair. Innovations (Phila). 2014;9(2):117–21; discussion 121.
20. Khanna G, Jaju A, Don S, Keys T, Hildebolt CF. Comparison of Haller index values calculated with chest radiographs versus CT for pectus excavatum evaluation. Pediatr Radiol. 2010;40(11):1763–7.
21. Mueller C, Saint-Vil D, Bouchard S. Chest x-ray as a primary modality for preoperative imaging of pectus excavatum. J Pediatr Surg. 2008;43(1):71–3.
22. Haller Jr JA, Kramer SS, Lietman SA. Use of CT scans in selection of patients for pectus excavatum surgery: a preliminary report. J Pediatr Surg. 1987; 22(10):904–6.
23. Haller Jr JA, Scherer LR, Turner CS, Colombani PM. Evolving management of pectus excavatum based on a single institutional experience of 664 patients. Ann Surg. 1989;209(5):578–82; discussion 582–3.
24. Albertal M, Vallejos J, Bellia G, Millan C, Rabinovich F, Buela E, Bignon H, Martinez-Ferro M. Changes in chest compression indexes with breathing underestimate surgical candidacy in patients with pectus excavatum: a computed tomography pilot study. J Pediatr Surg. 2013;48(10):2011–6.
25. Birkemeier KL, Podberesky DJ, Salisbury S, Serai S. Breathe in… breathe out… stop breathing: does phase of respiration affect the Haller index in patients with pectus excavatum? AJR Am J Roentgenol. 2011;197(5):W934–9.
26. St Peter SD, Juang D, Garey CL, Laituri CA, Ostlie DJ, Sharp RJ, Snyder CL. A novel measure for pectus excavatum: the correction index. J Pediatr Surg. 2011;46(12):2270–3.

27. Masaoka A, Kondo S, Sasaki S, Hara F, Mizuno T, Yamakawa Y, Kobayashi T, Fujii Y. Thirty years' experience of open-repair surgery for pectus excavatum: development of a metal-free procedure. Eur J Cardiothorac Surg. 2012;41(2):329–34.

28. Lee C, Park HJ, Lee S. New computerized tomogram (Ct) indices for pectus excavatum: tools for assessing modified techniques for asymmetry in Nuss repair. Chest. 2004;126(4_MeetingAbstracts):777S-a-777S.

29. Kim HC, Park HJ, Ham SY, Nam KW, Choi SY, Oh JS, Choi H, Jeong GS, Park SW, Kim MG, Sun K. Development of automatized new indices for radiological assessment of chest-wall deformity and its quantitative evaluation. Med Biol Eng Comput. 2008;46(8):815–23.

30. Chu ZG, Yu JQ, Yang ZG, Peng LQ, Bai HL, Li XM. Correlation between sternal depression and cardiac rotation in pectus excavatum: evaluation with helical CT. AJR Am J Roentgenol. 2010;195(1):W76–80.

31. Kim M, Lee KY, Park HJ, Kim HY, Kang EY, Oh YW, Seo BK, Je BK, Choi EJ. Development of new cardiac deformity indexes for pectus excavatum on computed tomography: feasibility for pre- and post-operative evaluation. Yonsei Med J. 2009;50(3):385–90.

32. Humphries CM, Anderson JL, Flores JH, Doty JR. Cardiac magnetic resonance imaging for perioperative evaluation of sternal eversion for pectus excavatum. Eur J Cardiothorac Surg. 2013;43(6):1110–3.

33. Marcovici PA, LoSasso BE, Kruk P, Dwek JR. MRI for the evaluation of pectus excavatum. Pediatr Radiol. 2011;41(6):757–8.

34. Lo Piccolo R, Bongini U, Basile M, Savelli S, Morelli C, Cerra C, Spinelli C, Messineo A. Chest fast MRI: an imaging alternative on pre-operative evaluation of pectus excavatum. J Pediatr Surg. 2012;47(3):485–9.

35. Birkemeier KL, Podberesky DJ, Salisbury S, Serai S. Limited, fast magnetic resonance imaging as an alternative for preoperative evaluation of pectus excavatum: a feasibility study. J Thorac Imaging. 2012;27(6):393–7.

36. Raichura N, Entwisle J, Leverment J, Beardsmore CS. Breath-hold MRI in evaluating patients with pectus excavatum. Br J Radiol. 2001;74(884):701–8.

37. Binazzi B, Innocenti Bruni G, Gigliotti F, Coli C, Romagnoli I, Messineo A, Lo Piccolo R, Scano G. Effects of the Nuss procedure on chest wall kinematics in adolescents with pectus excavatum. Respir Physiol Neurobiol. 2012;183(2):122–7.

38. Gürkan U, Aydemir B, Aksoy S, Akgöz H, Tosu AR, Öz D, Güngör B, Yılmaz H, Bolca O. Echocardiographic assessment of right ventricular function before and after surgery in patients with pectus excavatum and right ventricular compression. Thorac Cardiovasc Surg. 2014;62(3):231–5.

39. Rodrigues PL, Direito-Santos B, Moreira AH, Fonseca JC, Pinho AC, Rodrigues NF, Henriques-Coelho T, Correia-Pinto J, Vilaça JL. Variations of the soft tissue thicknesses external to the ribs in pectus excavatum patients. J Pediatr Surg. 2013;48(9):1878–86.

40. Poncet P, Kravarusic D, Richart T, Evison R, Ronsky JL, Alassiri A, Sigalet D. Clinical impact of optical imaging with 3-D reconstruction of torso topography in common anterior chest wall anomalies. J Pediatr Surg. 2007;42(5):898–903.

41. Lawson ML, Barnes-Eley M, Burke BL, Mitchell K, Katz ME, Dory CL, Miller SF, Nuss D, Croitoru DP, Goretsky MJ, Kelly Jr RE. Reliability of a standardized protocol to calculate cross-sectional chest area and severity indices to evaluate pectus excavatum. J Pediatr Surg. 2006;41(7):1219–25.

42. Nakahara K, Ohno K, Miyoshi S, Maeda H, Monden Y, Kawashima Y. An evaluation of operative outcome in patients with funnel chest diagnosed by means of the computed tomogram. J Thorac Cardiovasc Surg. 1987;93(4):577–82.

43. Kilda A, Basevicius A, Barauskas V, Lukosevicius S, Ragaisis D. Radiological assessment of children with pectus excavatum. Indian J Pediatr. 2007;74(2):143–7.

44. Kilda A, Lukosevicius S, Barauskas V, Jankauskaite Z, Basevicius A. Radiological changes after Nuss operation for pectus excavatum. Medicina (Kaunas). 2009;45(9):699–705.

45. Herrmann KA, Zech C, Strauss T, Hatz R, Schoenberg S, Reiser M. Cine MRI of the thorax in patients with pectus excavatum. Radiologe. 2006;46(4):309–16. German.

Traditional Treatment for Chest-Wall Deformities and Novel Treatment Methods

8

Natalie L. Simon and Shyam K. Kolvekar

Abstract

Traditional treatment for chest-wall deformities relies upon surgical inter-ventions that aim to increase thoracic function and restore kinetic and structural integrity to halt future chest-wall deformation prevent future deterioration of the chest wall. The Ravitch procedure is the most common intervention and involves subperichondrial resection of the deformed cos-tal cartilages and sternal osteotomy for fixation of the sternum anteriorly. Novel minimally invasive techniques are gaining popularity amongst cen-ters specialising in chest wall reconstruction, such as the Nuss procedure. At our centre we are researching the benefit of patient centered anesthesia on pain management post- Nuss procedure. We are also investigating vari-ous different techniques for bar removal and insertion using wire-assisted techniques. All of our research aims to increase the efficacy of minimally invasive corrective procedures.

Keywords

Chest wall deformity • Pectus Excavatum • Sternum • Malformation • Costal cartilages

N.L. Simon, MBBS
Department of School of Medical Education,
Kings College London, London, UK

S.K. Kolvekar, FRCSCTh (✉)
Department of Cardiothoracic Surgery,
University College London Hospitals, The Heart
Hospital and Barts Heart Center, London, UK
e-mail: kolvekar@yahoo.com

Ravitch Procedure

The Ravitch procedure is a primary intervention to correct pectus excavatum [1]. The technique involves a midline incision being made from the manubrium to epigastrium, under intratracheal anesthesia. A division at the lateral border of the deformity is made separating the lowermost car-tilages of either side and displacing them away from the sternum. This surgical technique may prove difficult in children as the perichondrium is not preserved and subperichondrial resection is difficult to perform. Following surgical resection of the cartilages, the xiphisternal articulation is separated, exposing the substernal ligament. This is then further divided and the xiphoid moves away from the sternum dividing any remaining rectus muscle attachments [2]. Pericostal sutures are situated onto the edges of the transverse osteotomy and ruffling sutures onto the perichondrium of resected cartilages. The full method used by Ravitch can be summarised below in four steps. Most methods of surgical correction of pectus excavatum include the basic steps described by Ravitch in 1949 [3].

1. Bilateral parasternal, and subperichondrial resection of the deformed costal cartilages
2. Detachment of the xiphoid process
3. Transverse wedge osteotomy at the upper edge of the sternal depression, and bending the sternum anteriorly to straighten its course
4. Securing the corrected position of the sternum

The following images will illustrate the steps involved in the Ravitch procedure, adapted from the original article [2]. Figure 8.1 shows the midline incision from manubrium to epigastrium. Here, the pectoral muscles are stripped back allowing for bilateral parasternal and subperichondrial resection of the deformed costal cartilages. Figure 8.2 shows how the surgeon gains access to the xiphoid, following division of the xiphisternal joint. Figure 8.3 illustrates the resection of costal cartilages and intercostal bundles on both sides allowing the sternum to be freed from its lower end. A transverse osteotomy is performed. The final stage, as shown in Fig. 8.4, is the elevation and the frac-

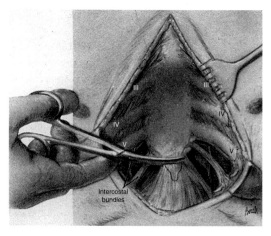

Fig. 8.2 How the surgeon gains access to the xiphoid, following division of the xiphisternal joint [2]

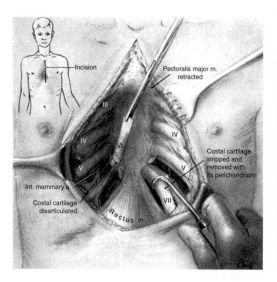

Fig. 8.1 The midline incision from manubrium to epigastrium. Here, the pectoral muscles are stripped back allowing for bilateral parasternal and subperichondrial resection of the deformed costal cartilages [2]

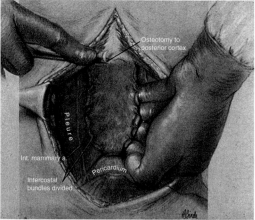

Fig. 8.3 Illustrates the resection of costal cartilages and intercostal bundles on both sides allowing the sternum to be freed from its lower end. A transverse osteotomy is performed [2]

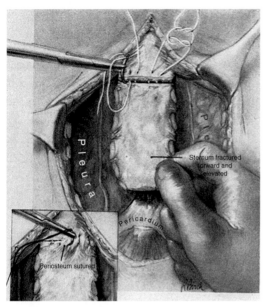

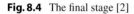

Fig. 8.4 The final stage [2]

turing of the posterior plate at the level of the transverse osteotomy. The new position is secured and maintained by mattress sutures and the periosteum is sutured [2].

Modification of Ravitch

Surgical repair of pectus excavatum relies on the corrected position of the sternum being maintained through the use of a sheet of synthetic mesh. Robicsek, 1978 presented a modification of the Ravitch procedure. This technique uses placement of Marlex mesh behind the sternum. The edge of the Marlex mesh is sutured to the peripheral stump of the resected ribs [3–5].

Following detachment of the xiphisternum, all loose mediastinal tissue is removed from the posterior sternum and the right pleural cavity drained with a chest tube, assuring optimal wound healing. The lower sternal end is bent forwards, breaking the posterior lamina at the transverse osteotomy. The Marlex mesh is spread tightly posterior to the sternum and has lateral

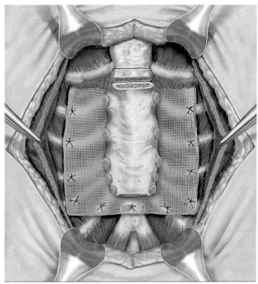

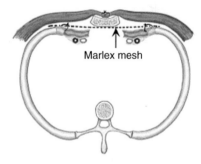

Fig. 8.5 Dr. Robicsek technique of Marlex mesh insertion to maintain the corrected position of the sternum

attachments to the remaining costal cartilages on their anterior side. The corrected position of sternum is now maintained and secured with the xiphoid process loosely attached to the lower end of mesh [3–5].

Figure 8.5 shows Dr. Robicsek technique of Marlex mesh insertion to maintain the corrected position of the sternum [3–5].

Comparative Studies

Recurrent pectus excavatum is experienced in a range of 2–37 % of patients having undergone corrective surgery for pectus excavatum.

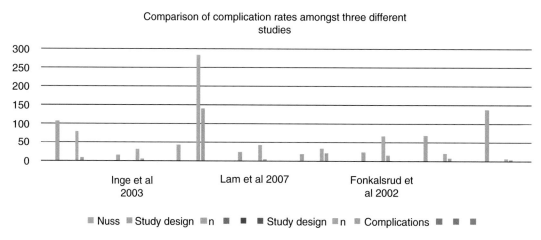

Fig. 8.6 Nuss procedure can be used in the corrective surgery of pectus carinatum. Two stabilisers are used to apply force to the sternum to depress the elevation and allow for fixation to the ribs on either side. This method is minimally invasive and does not require thoracoscopy (Adapted from Nasr et al. [1])

Table 8.1 Nuss procedure

	Jo et al. [10]		Inge et al. [11]		Lam et al. [12]		Fonkalsrud et al. [13]	
	Nuss	Ravitch	Nuss	Ravitch	Nuss	Ravitch	Nuss	Ravitch
Study design	**Retrospective**		**Retrospective**		**Retrospective**		**Retrospective**	
n	107	16	43	25	19	24	68	139
Complications	8	3	6	1	0	13	24	6
Reoperation	3	0	3	0	0	0	7	0
Duration of surgery (min)	67.2±33.1	196.9±61	70	198	72.1±19	84.1±24.9	75±21	212±37.5
Length of hospital stay (d)	8±1.6	15.9±2.3	2.4	4.4	4.5±0.9	3.9±0.7	6.5±0.75	2.9±0.75
Time to ambulation	6.3±0.9	12.9±3.6	–	–	3.8±1.1	2.7±0.8	–	–

	Miller et al. [14]		Nuss et al. [15]		Molik et al. [16]		Boehm et al. [17]	
	Nuss	Ravitch	Nuss	Ravitch	Nuss	Ravitch	Nuss	Ravitch
Study design	**Retrospective**		**Prospective**		**Retrospective**		**Retrospective**	
n	80	32	284	43	35	68	21	7
Complications	9	6	141	5	23	17	9	4
Reoperation	4	0	0	0	8	4	3	0
Duration of surgery	53	143	–	–	198	282	53±42.5	125±2.5
Length of hospital stay	3.7	3.2	–	–	4.8	4		–
Time to ambulation	–	–	–	–	–	–		

	Antonoff et al. [18]	
	Nuss	Ravitch
Study design	**Retrospective**	
n	14	56
Complications	5	8
Reoperation	0	1
Duration of surgery	109±8	110±4
Length of hospital stay	3.9±0.6	2.2±0.1
Time to ambulation	–	–

With permission from Nasr et al. [1]

Table 8.2 Specific complications

	Jo et al. [10]	Inge et al. [11]	Lam et al. [12]	Fonkalsrud et al. [13]	Miller et al. [14]	Nuss et al. [15]	Molik et al. [16]	Boehm et al. [17]	Antonoff et al. [18]	Sum
Reoperation										
Ravitch	0	0	0	0	0	0	4	0	3	7
Nuss	3	3	0	7	4	0	8	3	4	32
Pneumothorax										0
Ravitch	1	0	0	3	1	3	0	1	3	12
Nuss	5	0	0	7	2	12	1	2	1	30
Hemothorax										0
Ravitch	1	0	0	0	2	0	0	0	0	3
Nuss	4	0	0	0	1	0	0	1	0	6
Blood transfusion										0
Ravitch	0	0	0	0	1	0	0	0	0	1
Nuss	0	0	0	0	10	0	0	0	0	10

Adapted from Nasr et al. [1]

Common causes of recurrence include: asymmetric PE, perichondrium cartilage damage, limited space following retrosternal dissection, infection, improper fixation and early removal retrosternal plate [6]. The Ravitch procedure has few, yet potentially serious, complications. One of these is phrenic nerve injury. If there is laceration of the phrenic nerve, the patient has trouble breathing and suffers considerably more pain. Breathing regulation is altered. Phrenic nerve injury can be caused by direct trauma and 10 % of cases of phrenic nerve damage are caused by operative trauma. When diaphragm paralysis occurs, the patient may suffer type 2 respiratory failure and require mechanical assistance.

Complication rates between the Ravitch and the Nuss procedure are similar. Length of hospital stay or time to ambulation post-surgical procedure is also similar amongst the two groups and differs only minimally. The rate of reoperation due to bar movement and migration from site of placement was higher in the Nuss group. This is the main factor causing persistent deformation and worsening long term outcomes. Postoperative pneumothorax and hemothorax were also higher in the Nuss group, whereas duration of surgery was longer in the Ravitch procedure. Patient satisfaction is relatively high in both surgical procedures [1, 7, 8].

In addition, a modification of the Nuss procedure can be used in the corrective surgery of pectus carinatum. Two stabilisers are used to apply force to the sternum to depress the elevation and allow for fixation to the ribs on either side. This method is minimally invasive and does not require thoracoscopy (Fig. 8.6, Tables 8.1 and 8.2) [9].

References

1. Nasr A, Fecteau A, Wales PW. Comparison of the Nuss and the Ravitch procedure for pectus excavatum repair: a meta-analysis. J Pediatr Surg. 2010;45(5): 880–6.
2. Ravitch M. The operative treatment of pectus excavatum. Ann Surg. 1949;129:429–44.
3. Robicsek F. Surgical repair of pectus excavatum and carinatum. Semin Thorac Cardiovasc Surg. 2009;21(1): 64–75.
4. Robicsek F. Marlex mesh support for the correction of very severe and recurrent pectus excavatum. Coll Works Cardiopulm Dis. 1979;22:11–4.
5. Welch KJ. Satisfactory surgical correction of pectus excavatum deformity in childhood; a limited opportunity. J Thorac Surg. 1958;36(5):697–713.
6. Lucenic M, Janik M, Benej R, Garchar A, Juhos P. Surgical repair of recurrent pectus excavatum in adults and adolescents. Rozhl Chir. 2015;94(3):111–6.
7. Oncel M, Tezcan B, Akyol KG, Dereli Y, Sunam GS. Clinical experience of repair of pectus excavatum and carinatum deformities. Cardiovasc J Afr. 2013; 24(8):318–21.
8. Cobben JM, Oostra RJ, van Dijk FS. Pectus excavatum and carinatum. Eur J Med Genet. 2014;57(8):414–7.
9. Martinez-Ferro M. New approaches to pectus and other minimally invasive surgery in Argentina. J Pediatr Surg. 2010;45(1):19–27.

10. Jo WM, Choi YH, Sohn YS et al. Surgical treatment for pectus excavatum. J Korean Med Sci. 2003;18:360–4.
11. Inge TH, Owings E, Blewett CJ et al. Reduced hospitalization cost for patients with pectus excavatum treated using minimally invasive surgery. Surg Endosc. 2003;17:1609–13.
12. Lam MW, Klassen AF, Montgomery CJ et al. Quality-of-life outcomes after surgical correction of pectus excavatum: a comparison of the Ravitch and Nuss procedures. J Pediatr Surg. 2008;43:819–25.
13. Fonkalsrud EW, Beanes S, Hebra A et al. Comparison of minimally invasive and modified Ravitch pectus excavatum repair. J Pediatr Surg. 2002;37:413–17.
14. Miller KA, Woods RK, Sharp RJ et al. Minimally invasive repair of pectus excavatum: a single institution's experience. Surgery. 2001;130:652–57.
15. Nuss D, Kelly Jr RE et al. A 10-year review of a minimally invasive technique for the correction of pectus excavatum. J Pediatr Surg. 1998;33:545–55.
16. Molik KA, Engum SA, Rescorla FJ et al. Pectus excavatum repair: experience with standard and minimal invasive techniques. J Pediatr Surg. 2001;36:324–28.
17. Boehm RA, Muensterer OJ, Till H. Comparing minimally invasive funnel chest repair versus the conventional technique: an outcome analysis in children. Plast Reconstr Surg. 2004;114:668–73.
18. Antonoff MB, Erickson AE, Hess DJ et al. When patients choose: comparison of Nuss, Ravitch, and Leonard procedures for primary repair of pectus excavatum. J Pediatr Surg. 2009;44:1113–18.

Minimal Invasive Repair of Pectus Excavatum

Hans K. Pilegaard

Abstract

The modern era of correction of pectus excavatum (PE) started in 1949 by Ravitch. Since several modifications to the technique were published, but it was the standard way to correct PE for long time. Prof Nuss's minimally technique changed the strategy for correction and seems now to be the standard technique for surgeons who correct PE. The optimal age for surgery is discussed. Most surgeons prefer that the patient is in the beginning of the puberty so the bar system is in situ through the growth spurt. It looks like that this decreases the recurrence rate. At this age the patients are also aware of the restrictions which are in the beginning of the treatment. But recently it has been offered to patient up to 40 years of age. Bar removal is done 3 years after correction and is a day surgery project. In most cases it is only necessary to open the incision where you have the stabilizer if you use the short bar technique. The complication are few in experienced hands. Most of the patients get a very beautiful result and are very satisfied with the operation.

Keywords

Pectus Excavtum • NUSS procedure • Sternal Bar

The modern era of correction of pectus excavatum (PE) started in 1949 where Ravitch published the his first paper [1]. Since several modifications to the technique were published, but it was the standard way to correct PE until Nuss orally presented his first work in 1997 and published it in 1998 [2]. This minimally technique changed the strategy for correction and seems now to be the standard technique for surgeons who correct PE. This paper dealed with 45 patients who were corrected through a 10-years course. The age group was from 1 to 15 years and at that time it was thought that the technique could only be used in children

H.K. Pilegaard, MD
Associate Professor, Department of Cardiothoracic and Vascular Surgery, Department of Clinical Medicine, Aarhus University Hospital, Denmark, Aarhus, Denmark
e-mail: pilegaard@dadlnet.dk

and adolescents because the rigidity of the chest in adults was too high. With the growing experience of the technique it has been shown that even patients in the fifties and sixties might be corrected by the Nuss-procedure [3, 4]. The original technique prescribed that the bar length should be from the mid axillary line on each side. The first operations were done without scope assistance but to make the intervention safer using of the thoracoscope is now mandatory. One of the problems with the technique was the risk of rotation of the bar. This was reduced by first adding a stabilizer, then fixing the stabilizer to the bar and finally using several circumcostal sutures around the bar and rib on the opposite site of the stabilizer. These reduced the risk from around 15 to 1 % [5]. Later the use of a shorter bar has been published and this change has shown the same low risk of rotation [6, 7]. Using the shorter bar is easier, using shorter time in the OR, gives the same good cosmetic result and is as stable as using the long original bar.

Indication for Surgery

In most published papers the indication for surgery is cosmetic complaints from the patient [8]. It has been known for many years that the patients too have several physiological symptoms [9] and recent studies have shown that correction without increasing the patients quality of life significantly [10–16] also means better movement of the chest [17, 18] and better cardiac performance [19, 20]. Some surgeons prefer to measure the Haller index, which should normally be bigger than 3.25 to indicate surgery, but the problem with the Haller index is that it is also depending of the chest shape, if it is flat or barrel shaped.

Surgery

The optimal age for surgery is discussed. Most surgeons prefer that the patient is in the beginning of the puberty so the bar system is in situ through the growth spurt. It looks like that this decreases the recurrence rate. At this age the patients are also aware of the restrictions which are in the beginning of the treatment. In girls I prefer that the there is some demarcation of the breasts so the incisions might be placed in the sulcus.

The surgery is done in general anaesthesia and prior to surgery an epidural catheter is placed to facilitate the postoperative pain treatment. Position of the patient is on the back either with the arms abducted or the arm along the body with a pillow behind the back [21] or in my mind better with the right arm elevated in front of the head to allow free movement of the scope. The deepest point is defined and the points for penetration of the chest wall are marked on the skin. These points should be just medially to the highest areas. The length of the bar should be so the right end covers two ribs and the left end is long enough to carry the stabilizer, so the stabilizer is placed very close to the hinge point. This gives a very stable system with a very limited risk of rotation. This means that the bar is placed asymmetric in the patient. The tunnel under the sternum is done guided by the scope which normally is only used from the right side. It is very important that the introducer is in close contact with the backside of the chest, if this is not true so you have to use an introducer with a longer tip. A template is bended to the expected shape of the chest after correction with some overcorrection 1–2 cm because the pressure from the sternum will cause some debending of the bar. The bar might be guided through the chest by a normal suture or a tape. The bar is inserted as an U and turned 180°. In most cases it might be done with the use of only one flipper.

Most of the patients only need one bar, which normally should support the sternum under the deepest point. The number of bars is depended on the length of the PE, the deepness and the rigidity of the chest wall. Around 30 % needs more than one bar. In many cases two bars might be inserted through the same incisions. In some cases an oblique bar gives a better cosmetic result. All bars are normally stabilized on the left side with a stabilizer, which is fixed either by a steel wire around the bar or an additional bending of the end.

The lung is expanded at the end of the operation by using a chest tube under water seal and is removed at the end of the operation.

An x-ray is done the second postoperative day before discharge. X-ray just after surgery is normally not required [22].

Pain Treatment

The pain treatment is a combination of epidural analgesia and perorally treatment. The epidural catheter is closed the second postoperative day in the morning. The day of the operation the patient have morphine and bupivacaine and the next day it is changed to pure bupivacaine. The first postoperative day the patient starts NSAID, Ibuprofen and often oxycodone. The oxycodone is stopped after 10–14 days, Ibuprofen and NSAID are normally stopped after 4 and 5 weeks postoperatively, respectively.

Postoperative Restrictions

The first 6 weeks the patients are not allowed to carry more than 2 kg in front of the body and 5 kg on the their back. They must not bike, not rotate the upper body more than 15° and should sleep on the back. Sleeping on the back is often the most difficult issue, giving the patient serious backpain, but most of the patients start spontaneously to turn in the bed after 5–7 weeks and then the backpain problems disappear.

In all 3 years heavy contact sport such as American football, rugby, icehockey and self-defence sports should be avoided.

Postoperative Follow-Up

The patients are seen in the outpatient clinic after 6 weeks for a clinical examination and an x-ray to see the position of the bar system. After this the patient is called 3 years later for bar removal. Should there be any problems in the mean time they may call the department.

Bar Removal

Bar removal is done 3 years after correction and is a day surgery project [23]. In most cases it is only necessary to open the incision where you have the stabilizer if you use the short bar technique [23].

Results

Most of the patients get a very beautiful result and are very satisfied with the operation. The complication are few in experienced hands.

References

1. Ravitch MM. The operative treatment of pectus excavatum. Ann Surg. 1949;129:429–44.
2. Nuss D, Kelly Jr RE, Croitoru DP, Katz ME. A 10-year review of a minimally invasive technique for the correction of pectus excavatum. J Pediatr Surg. 1998;33:545–52.
3. Pilegaard HK, Licht PB. Routine use of minimally invasive surgery for pectus excavatum in adults. Ann Thorac Surg. 2008;86:952–6.
4. Pilegaard HK. Extending the use of Nuss procedure in patients older than 30 years. Eur J Cardiothorac Surg. 2011;40:334–7.
5. Nuss D. Recent experiences with minimally invasive pectus excavatum repair "Nuss procedure". Jpn J Thorac Cardiovasc Surg. 2005;53:338–44.
6. Pilegaard HK, Licht PB. Early results following the Nuss operation for pectus excavatum – a single-institution experience of 383 patients. Interact Cardiovasc Thorac Surg. 2008;7:54–7.
7. Pilegaard HK, Licht PB. Can absorbable stabilizers be used routinely in the Nuss procedure? Eur J Cardiothorac Surg. 2009;35:561–4.
8. Krasopoulos G, Goldstraw P. Minimally invasive repair of pectus excavatum deformity. Eur J Cardiothorac Surg. 2010.
9. Kelly Jr RE. Pectus excavatum: historical background, clinical picture, preoperative evaluation and criteria for operation. Semin Pediatr Surg. 2008;17:181–93.
10. Roberts J, Hayashi A, Anderson JO, Martin JM, Maxwell LL. Quality of life of patients who have undergone the Nuss procedure for pectus excavatum: preliminary findings. J Pediatr Surg. 2003;38:779–83.
11. Lawson ML, Cash TF, Akers R, Vasser E, Burke B, Tabangin M, Welch C, Croitoru DP, Goretsky MJ, Nuss D, Kelly Jr RE. A pilot study of the impact of surgical repair on disease-specific quality of life

among patients with pectus excavatum. J Pediatr Surg. 2003;38:916–8.

12. Krasopoulos G, Dusmet M, Ladas G, Goldstraw P. Nuss procedure improves the quality of life in young male adults with pectus excavatum deformity. Eur J Cardiothorac Surg. 2006;29:1–5.

13. Metzelder ML, Kuebler JF, Leonhardt J, Ure BM, Petersen C. Self and parental assessment after minimally invasive repair of pectus excavatum: lasting satisfaction after bar removal. Ann Thorac Surg. 2007;83:1844–9.

14. Kelly Jr RE, Cash TF, Shamberger RC, Mitchell KK, Mellins RB, Lawson ML, Oldham K, Azizkhan RG, Hebra AV, Nuss D, Goretsky MJ, Sharp RJ, Holcomb 3rd GW, Shim WK, Megison SM, Moss RL, Fecteau AH, Colombani PM, Bagley T, Quinn A, Moskowitz AB. Surgical repair of pectus excavatum markedly improves body image and perceived ability for physical activity: multicenter study. Pediatrics. 2008;122: 1218–22.

15. Lam MW, Klassen AF, Montgomery CJ, LeBlanc JG, Skarsgard ED. Quality-of-life outcomes after surgical correction of pectus excavatum: a comparison of the Ravitch and Nuss procedures. J Pediatr Surg. 2008; 43:819–25.

16. Jacobsen EB, Thastum M, Jeppesen JH, Pilegaard HK. Health-related quality of life in children and adolescents undergoing surgery for pectus excavatum. Eur J Pediatr Surg. 2010;20:85–91.

17. Redlinger Jr RE, Kelly RE, Nuss D, Goretsky M, Kuhn MA, Sullivan K, Wootton AE, Ebel A, Obermeyer RJ. Regional chest wall motion dysfunction in patients with pectus excavatum demonstrated via optoelectronic plethysmography. J Pediatr Surg. 2011;46:1172–6.

18. Redlinger Jr RE, Wootton A, Kelly RE, Nuss D, Goretsky M, Kuhn MA, Obermeyer RJ. Optoelectronic plethysmography demonstrates abrogation of regional chest wall motion dysfunction in patients with pectus excavatum after Nuss repair. J Pediatr Surg. 2012;47: 160–4.

19. Lesbo M, Tang M, Nielsen HH, Frokiaer J, Lundorf E, Pilegaard HK, Hjortdal VE. Compromised cardiac function in exercising teenagers with pectus excavatum. Interact Cardiovasc Thorac Surg. 2011;13:377–80.

20. Maagaard M, Tang M, Ringgaard S, Nielsen HH, Frokiaer J, Haubuf M, Pilegaard HK, Hjortdal VE. Normalized cardiopulmonary exercise function in patients with pectus excavatum three years after operation. Ann Thorac Surg. 2013;96:272–8.

21. de Campos JR, Fonseca MH, Werebe Ede C, Velhote MC, Jatene FB. Technical modification of the Nuss operation for the correction of pectus excavatum. Clinics (Sao Paulo). 2006;61:185–6.

22. Knudsen MR, Nyboe C, Hjortdal VE, Pilegaard HK. Routine postoperative chest X-ray is unnecessary following the Nuss procedure for pectus excavatum. Interact Cardiovasc Thorac Surg. 2013;16:830–3.

23. Nyboe C, Knudsen MR, Pilegaard HK. Elective pectus bar removal following Nuss procedure for pectus excavatum: a single-institution experience. Eur J Cardiothorac Surg. 2011;39:1040–2.

Personal Experience in Minimally Invasive Treatment of Pectus Carinatum

Mustafa Yuksel

Abstract

Pectus Carinatum is the second mostly encountered congenital chest wall deformity following Pectus Excavatum. Deformity becomes apparent during puberty, due to active growth; which leads to cosmetic and psychosocial problems. "Minimally Invasive Repair of Pectus Carinatum" gained popularity among surgeons during last decade. In this chapter, we try to explain surgical details, preoperative and postoperative workup period of the deformity. We also present our whole experience about correction of pectus carinatum.

Keywords

Chest wall deformity • Pectus Carinatum • Minimally Invasive • Personal Experience • Operation Technique

Pectus Carinatum (PC) is the second mostly encountered congenital chest wall deformity following Pectus Excavatum (PE). It is characterized by convex protrusion of costal cartilages, anterior chest wall and sternum. PC is classified into two subgroups as "chondrogladiolar" and "condromanubrial" according to the anatomic location of protrusion. Chondrogladiolar deformity is defined as asymmetric or symmetric protrusion of inferior costal cartilages and corpus sternum. Asymmetric deformity results due to

unilateral overgrowth of costal cartilages and rotation of the sternum. In chondromanubrial deformity, manubrium sterni and superior costal cartilages are protruded. Due to this arched appearance, the deformity is named as "pectus arcuatum". Pectus arcuatum is less than 1 % of all PC cases [1]. Surgical treatment for Pectus Arcuatum is modified Ravitch Sternoplasty.

Although the etiology of PC is unclear, 25 % of the patients have positive family history for chest wall deformity which supports genetic inheritance [2]. Before 11 years of age, prominent protrusion of PC is seen only less than 10 % of the patients. Deformity becomes apparent during puberty, due to active growth; which leads to cosmetic and psychosocial problems during this period [3].

M. Yuksel, MD, PhD
Department of Thoracic Surgery, Marmara University Hospital, Istanbul, Turkey
e-mail: drmustafayuksel@gmail.com

PC is encountered at a ratio of 1:5 compared to PE patients, seen four times more in males than females [2]. It is more popular among Hispanic population but rare in Asian and African population. PC can be seen solely by itself, as well as it may be a part of genetic disorders like Marfan Syndrome, trisomy 18, homocsytinuria, Morque Syndrome, Ehlers-Danlos Syndrome. PC may accompany some congenital heart diseases and connective tissue disorders as well. Scoliosis is the most concomitant anomaly of the skeletal system at a ratio of 15 % [2–4].

Most of the PC patients are asymptomatic but frequent symptoms are shortness of breath, fatigue, pain over the deformity [5]. Indication for the operation is based on cosmetic and psychosocial problems.

Surgical Treatment of PC

At the beginning of twenty-first century, the treatment for PE shifted towards "minimally invasive repair of pectus excavatum (MIRPE) known as "Nuss procedure". It was performed successfully using an easy technique. Standard surgical procedure for correction of PC was Ravitch sternoplasty. Several modifications had been applied and performed until 2005 [6–8]. Abramson defined a modification of Nuss procedure to be used for PC in 2005. It is named as "Minimally Invasive Repair of Pectus Carinatum". In this technique known as MIRPC, the sternum is compressed by implanting a metal bar in the prester-

nal region and securing it bilaterally to the posterolateral portion of the costal arches [9, 10].

Decision Making for the Treatment (Treatment Type)

Ideal age for correction of the deformity is between 14 and 18 years old. We perform "compression test" preoperatively for the assessment of treatment type. The patient in upright position leans upon the wall, we apply compression to the maximum protruding region of the chest by "compression test device" which we developed (Fig. 10.1), and measure the pressure correcting the deformity. If the pressure is less than 10 kg, the patient is appropriate for orthosis treatment. Between 10 and 25 kg the patients are considered to be appropriate for MIRPC. If the pressure is over 25 kg, Ravitch sternoplasty is the choice of surgical treatment [11, 12].

Orthosis Treatment

If the pressure test results are less than 10 kg, the patients may benefit from (compressive) orthotic bracing which generally lasts 6 months. The patients have to wear custom-made orthotic brace all the day through (Fig. 10.2). Orthosis is suggested for children older than 5 years old due to the problem of coherence. If the deformity persists more than 6 months, orthosis therapy may prolong for 9–12 months.

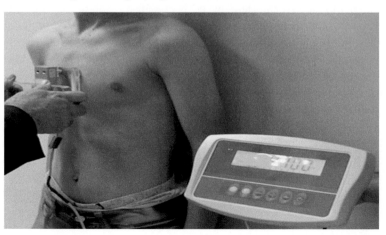

Fig. 10.1 Measuring the pressure correcting the deformity by the help of "compression test device"

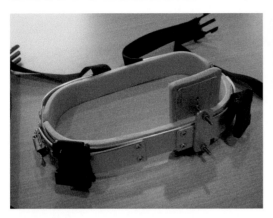

Fig. 10.2   Custom-made orthotic brace

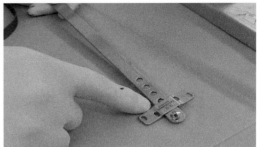

Fig. 10.3   Bar and stabilizer of pectus carinatum

Preoperative Evaluation and Preparation

Postero-anterior and lateral chest radiograms and photos of the patient in six different angles of the thoracic cavity are taken. Routine laboratory analysis, ECG and pulmonary function tests are performed. We do not routinely perform echocardiography and thoracic computed tomography unless complicated anomalies are suspected.

The bar used for MIRPC operation is metalic composition of nickel and steel (Fig. 10.3). If the patient is allergenic for metals, it is not appropriate to use this bar. In these kind of cases, we prefer inserting titanium bars instead of standard ones. Detailed patient history and allergy skin test is useful for identifying the metal allergy. We order special titanium bars for the allergenic patients [13–16].

Surgical Technique

Patients are positioned in supine position with both arms abducted and then are entubated by single lumen tracheal tube. Maximal protrusion area is the path of the bar. Mid-axillary lines, where edges of the bar will be placed bilaterally, is identified with marker pen. Mid-axillary lines will also be marked for the right place of the stabilizers. The length of the bar is designated according to this

path. Templates (aluminium models) are used for designating the proper bar size. We compress the chest wall until the desired appearance is obtained. The carinatum bar, which is in same size with the model, is formed according to template. After bending the carinatum bar, the surgeon starts with 3 cm long incisions on mid-axillary lines bilaterally and prepares space for stabilizers under serratus anterior muscle. After dissection of the muscles, two parallel ribs are chosen where stabilizers will be fixed by the help of the hook. One centimeter incision is made on the periosteum of the chosen ribs and the periosteum is dissected. A hook is placed around the rib subperiostally and a suction catheter is attached to the tip of the hook and the hook is pulled back with the catheter (Fig. 10.4). A sternal cable (Pioneer Sternal Cable System, Marquette, MI) (if unavailable, two to three times folded no: 5 steel wire) is passed through the suction catheter which is around the rib using it as a guide for fixing the stabilizer. This procedure is repeated on both sides on each ribs. When wrapping up with the wires are completed, stabilizers are fixed to ribs. Long aortic clamps are used to make tunnel under the muscles for the insertion of the bar. Then introducer is inserted through tunnel. By the help of the introducer, a 28 Fr thorax drain is passed through the tunnel as a guide. The bar is attached to the drain and both are pulled back from the tunnel. The bar is placed into the tunnel over the sternum and the edges are slipped into the stabilizer. Bar is fixed to the stabilizer in proper position by the help of clips (Fig. 10.5). 2/0 vicryl sutures are used to cover the muscle fibers over the stabilizers and edges of the bar. Subcutaneus tissue is

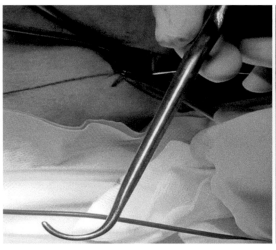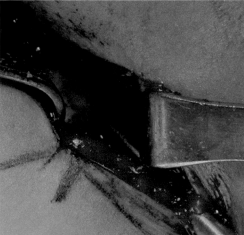

Fig. 10.4 Hook used to turn around (girdle) the rib

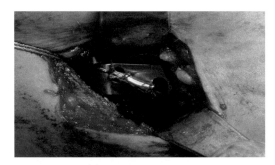

Fig. 10.5 Fixing the stabilizer to the ribs by wires

closed continuously by 2/0 vicryl and cutaneous tissue by 5/0 monocryl sutures.

Postoperative Period

Pain is the most serious problem just after the operation. Pain is due to stabilizers, which are placed subperiostally with wires, can be relieved with intravenous (iv) analgesics. IV "Patient Controlled Analgesia (PCA)" is the preferred method for these patients.

Patients are mobilized 6 h after the operation. Analgesics are terminated on 3rd or 4th postoperative day and discharged with oral analgesics on 5th day. Patients can go back to school or work after 2–3 weeks rest at home. It is advised to lie back for the first month and participate in active sports for 3 months.

Early and Late Complications

Pneumothorax and wound infection are the most frequent complications in early postoperative period. Physicians operating MIRPC always have to keep in mind that surgery is based on implanting foreign body into the patient. Antibiotherapy for prophylaxis and postoperative period with close care reduces infection rates less than %1 [17].

If secondary infection occurs, it can be treated by drainage, proper antibiotherapy and even in some serious cases removal of the bar may be necessary.

Late complications are basically breakage of wires that are holding the stabilizers, infection, erosion of the skin, hyperpigmentation, late allergic reactions, cutaneous adhesion and insufficient correction.

Wire breakage is an important late complication as well. We can make two or three fold spiral wires to prevent this complication. In our series we used sternal cable (Pioneer Sternal Cable System, Marquette, MI) and avoided the risk afterwards.

Proper patient selection, respiratory physiotherapy, prophylactic antibiotherapy and most importantly progress with experience in the operation have great benefit on decreasing complications.

Results

Results for MIRPC in long lasting period is almost satisfactory on different series [18]. In our series of 140 cases, questionnarie of patient satisfaction was perfect except three patients.

Removal/Withdrawal of the Bar

At the end of the period, bar is removed under general anesthesia. Bar and stabilizers are exposed by using former incisions. Clips of the bar are taken away and wires which connect the stabilizers and ribs are cut with wire cutters. Initially the wires and then the stabilizers are removed. Curve of the bar is straightened on one edge by specially made bar-twister and the bar is pulled carefully by the hooks from the other edge.

Marmara University Experience

The standard PE bars were used in MIRPC operation for the first three cases. Since 2008, we use bar and stabilizer systems which we invented for MIRPC.

Between January 2006-November 2014, in approximately 8 years, we performed 140 MIRPC for Pectus Carinatum patients (Figs. 10.6, 10.7, and 10.8)

122 of 140 patients were male and ages ranged between 10 and 33 years with a median age of 16.5. In all patients, indication was cosmetic problems leading to anxiety and psychosocial problems.

Thirteen cases had family history of congenital chest wall deformities (PE or PC). All of the 140 cases, who are chondrogladioler type pectus carinatum deformity, underwent MIRPC operation with one bar and two stabilizers. Operation lasted 45–110 min (median: 60 min). Length of stay was 2–10 days with a median of 5 days.

Most frequent early complication was pneumothorax in 12 cases. Three of them were treated with tube thoracostomy, another two with pleural catheter and the rest had resorbed spontaneously.

We have experienced wire breakage in the early postoperative period in three cases who were operated with single layer steel wires (twice wire breakage in one case), erosion of the skin in three cases, wound infection in nine cases and severe pain in one patient as most frequent complications. The patients with wire breakage underwent another operation where two to three

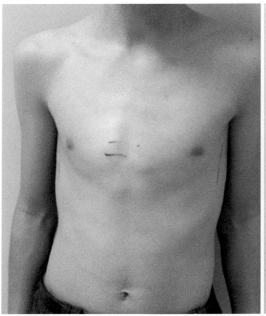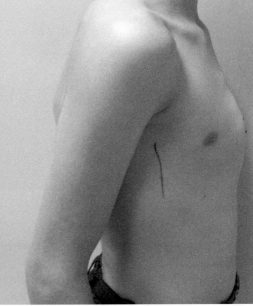

Fig. 10.6   14-year-old male with symmetric Pectus Carinatum deformity

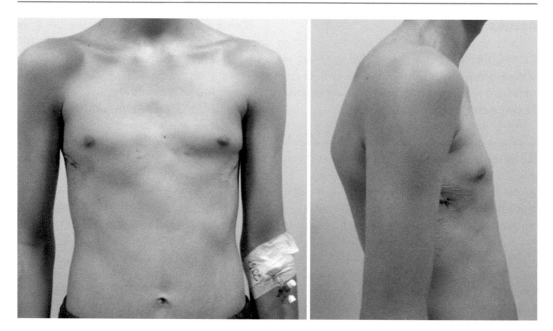

Fig. 10.7 Postoperative day

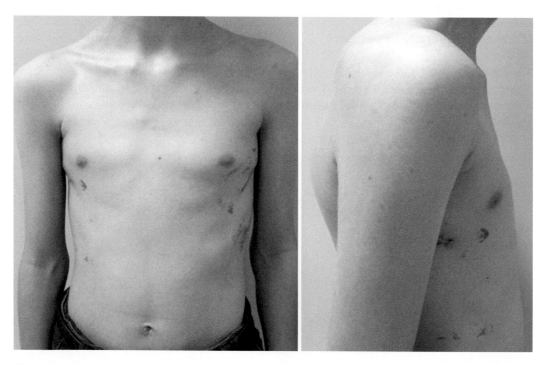

Fig. 10.8 Postoperative 2nd week

layered spiral wires were replaced with broken ones.

Patients with dermal erosion were reoperated for revision of the skin. Patients with wound infection were treated with appropriate antibiot-

ics. One of our patients who had been operated using standard PE bar had severe pain that analgesics could not resolve. As a result of this complication we had to remove the bar 5 months after the operation.

Wound infection and overcorrection are the leading late postoperative complications with 9 and 7 patients respectively. Wire breakage (6 patients), Nickel allergy (5 patients), hyperpigmentation (3 patients) and cutting of the ribs by sternal cable (2 patients) are the other late complications.

Up to date: we had removed bars of 60 patients among our series after a follow-up of 2–3 years. All of them were removed without any complication on the basis of routine procedure. Recurrence occurred only in two patients after the operations and we followed up these patients with orthosis. With the use of modified bars, we remove bars within 2 years after MIRPC.

Patient satisfaction surveys showed all scores were higher at postoperative 6th month except one patient. four cases were not satisfied with the results. Both psychosocial and physical change were significant. Patients were more positive, more compatible with self-confidence and more social after the operation. Overall patient satisfaction after MIRPC operation was 96 %.

Conclusion

According to our 8 years of experience and conservative experience of other centers expressed that MIRPC is a minimally invasive technique with shorter operation time, low morbidity and has almost perfect satisfactory results. This technique is very successful for correcting PC deformities and improving quality of life. In the light of these data, MIRPC should be the treatment of choice for Pectus Carinatum patients.

References

1. Shamberger RC, Welch KJ. Surgical correction of chondromanubrial deformity (Currarino Silverman syndrome). J Pediatr Surg. 1988;23:319–22.
2. Golladay ES. Pectus carinatum and other deformities of the chest wall. In: Ziegler MM, Azizkhan RG, Weber TR, editors. Operative pediatric surgery. New York: McGraw-Hill; 2003. p. 269–77.
3. Fonkalsrud EW, Beanes S. Management of pectus carinatum: 30 years experience. World J Surg. 2001;25:898–903.
4. Saxena AK, Willital GH. Surgical repair of pectus carinatum. Int Surg. 1999;4:326–30.
5. Fonkalsrud EW, Anselmo DM. Less extensive techniques for repair of pectus carinatum: the undertreated chest deformity. J Am Coll Surg. 2004;198:898–905.
6. Nuss D, Kelly Jr RE, Croitoru DP, Katz ME. A 10-year review of a minimally invasive technique for the correction of pectus excavatum. J Pediatr Surg. 1988;33:545–52.
7. Abramson H. A minimally invasive technique to repair pectus carinatum. Preliminary report. Arch Bronconeumol. 2005;41:349–51.
8. Ravitch M. The operative correction of pectus carinatum (pigeon breast). Ann Surg. 1960;151:705–14.
9. Abramson H, D'Agostino J, Wuscovi S. A 5-year experience with a minimally invasive technique for pectus carinatum repair. J Pediatr Surg. 2009;44:118–23.
10. Yüksel M, Bostancı K, Evman S. Minimally invasive repair of pectus carinatum using a newly designed bar and stabilizer: a single-institution experience. Eur J Cardiothorac Surg. 2011. doi:10.1016/j.ejcts.2010.11.047 [Basımda].
11. Robicsek F, Watts LT, Fokin AA. Surgical repair of pectus excavatum and carinatum. Semin Thorac Cardiovasc Surg. 2009;21:64–75.
12. Yüksel M, Bostancı K, Eldem B. Stabilizing the sternum using an absorbable copolymer plate after open surgery for pectus deformities. Multimed Man Cardiothorac Surg. 2011. doi:10.1510/mmcts.2010.004879.
13. Nuss D. Minimally invasive surgical repair of pectus excavatum. Semin Pediatr Surg. 2008;17(3):209–17.
14. Rushing GD, Goretsky MJ, Gustin T, et al. When it is not an infection: metal allergy after the Nuss procedure for repair of pectus excavatum. J Pediatr Surg. 2007;42(1):93–7.
15. Pilegaard HK, Licht PB. Can absorbable stabilizers be used routinely in the Nuss procedure? Eur J Cardiothorac Surg. 2009;35:561–4.
16. Vlkel W, Pabst F, Klemm E. The use of resorbable osteosynthesis materials. Laryngorhinootologie. 2011; 90:23–5.
17. Calkins CM, Shew SB, Sharp RJ, et al. Management of postoperative infections after the minimally invasive pectus repair. J Pediatr Surg. 2005;40:1004–8.
18. Jaroszewski D, Fonkalsrud EW. Repair of pectus chest deformities in 320 adult patients: 21 year experience. Ann Thorac Surg. 2007;84:429–33.

Pain Management in the Surgical Correction of Chest Wall Deformities

11

Elizabeth M.C. Ashley

Abstract

The thoracoscopic placement of Nuss pectus bars for the correction of pectus excavatum is a painful procedure., which poses a challenge for the thoracic anaesthetist. Adequate pain management can expedite post-operative recovery and reduce complications. It may also prevent the development of chronic post-operative pain. Previously thoracic epidural analgesia has been favoured by centres in North America and Europe, but there is tendency to move away from this in favour of a multimodal approach to analagesia, including regional blockade, opiate infusions and patient-controlled analagesia, with non-steroidal anti-inflammatory drugs, paracetamol and other novel analgesics given in addition for their synergistic and opiate sparing effects

Keywords

Multi-modal analgesia • Opiates • Patient-Controlled Analagesia • Non-steriodal anti-inflammatory drugs • Novel agents • Regional Blockade • Thoracic Epidurals • Post-operative Care

Surgical Procedures

Surgery for the correction of chest wall deformities, the commonest of which is pectus excavatum, is becoming more frequently performed, as minimally invasive surgical techniques are developed. This poses a challenge for the thoracic anaesthetist to provide appropriate perioperative pain relief for thoracic surgery for benign disease and what in many cases is an ostensibly cosmetic procedure.

Pectus correction was originally carried out by the Ravitch procedure. This was major thoracic surgery, involving removal of costal-cartilages and elevation of the sternum using small steel bars. This has now been super-ceded by the Nuss procedure. The Nuss procedure involves the thoracoscopic placement of a concave pectus bar, from the right side of the chest which is placed

E.M.C. Ashley, BSc, MBChB, FRCA, FFICM
Department of Anesthesia and Cardiothoracic
Intensive Care, The Heart Hospital UCLH,
London, UK
e-mail: elizabethashley@doctors.org.uk

beneath the intercostal muscles and then flipped into a convex position to elevate the sternum, within the chest. The procedure involves two small (approximately 2 cm) lateral incisions in the chest wall for each pectus bar. One or two bars are used during each corrective procedure [1]. Severity of pain is related to the severity of the pectus (greater Haller Index) and the amount of elevation that is required. Two bars are paradoxically often less painful than one.

The bars are removed after approximately 2 years. This involves a second anaesthetic and further perioperative pain management.

Other procedures for chest wall surgery include local plastic reconstructive surgery, plastic flaps and silicone implants.

The patient population is predominantly young males with body image issues or perceived shortness of breath on exertion due to restrictive lung function. They are generally a highly-motivated group, who actively seek out the surgery and surgeons and are therefore motivated and prepared for a degree of post-operative pain.

However, the surgery is extremely painful and inadequate pain management can exacerbate post-operative complications, cause bar displacement, limit early mobilisation, limit enhanced-recovery and prolong hospital stay.

There is also an incidence of chronic post-operative pain and the patient should be aware of this before undergoing the procedure.

Intra-operative Pain Management

The pain management options include thoracic epidural anaesthesia or an opiate based technique. Regional blocks also play a role.

A survey and review of pain management following Nuss procedure was carried out over 108 Paediatric Hospitals in North America, Europe, Asia and Australasia, and was published in 2014. Fifty-five institutions carrying out the NUSS procedure responded and were performing the operations on patients aged between 14 and 17 years of age. Ninety-one percent of institutions used thoracic epidural anaesthesia and otherwise intravenous patient-controlled analgesia was used.

Sixteen percent of the paediatric hospitals said they were stopping epidurals, preferring opiate PCAs [2]. A meta-analysis comparing epidural analgesia and Intravenous patient-controlled analgesia was also published in 2014. Only three randomised-controlled trials and three retrospective studies met inclusion criteria. Epidural analgesia produced slightly lower pain scores immediately post-operatively and in the first 12–48 h post-surgery, compared with PCA, but this did not translate into significantly different secondary outcomes such as reduced length of hospital stay and reduced hospital costs [3].

Opiates

A standard anaesthetic technique involves a small dose of a short-acting opiate on induction of anaesthesia, such as fentanyl, followed by a longer-acting opiate such as morphine during the procedure. Immediate post-operative pain can be managed in the recovery room using protocolised incremental doses of intravenous fentanyl or morphine administered by recovery nurses, with assiduous respiratory monitoring, and sedation scoring, until the patient is comfortable.

Patient-Controlled Opiate Analgesia

Patient controlled opiate anaesthesia (PCA) with fentanyl or morphine is used in the post-operative period. Many studies report using PCA in addition to epidural analgesia. This requires careful monitoring of cardiovascular and neurological observations. Opiates should not be given via two different routes, i.e. by intravenous PCA and epidural infusion, to avoid opiate side effects. In younger children nurse controlled analgesia (NCA) can be used. This involves regular pain assessments by the nursing-staff, with a nurse-administered opiate bolus based on the patient's weight. A standard adult PCA protocol includes a bolus dose (e.g. 1 mg of morphine or 20 ug of fentanyl) and a 5 minute lockout period, with or without a low dose background infusion. This enables the patient to titrate opiate consumption according to his or her individual requirements and expectations of post-operative pain. More severe pectus is associated with higher PCA morphine consumption. There was an increase in 6 % morphine usage with every 1 cm increase in pectus depth [4].

Non-steroidal Anti-inflammatory Drugs

Intra-operative opiate analgesia can be supplemented by drugs with different mechanisms of action, which act synergistically and have an opiate-sparing effect. Conventional non-steroidal anti-inflammatory drugs (Cox-1 inhibitors) that can be administered intravenously include diclofenac and ketorolac. They inhibit the cyclooxygenase system and prostaglandin synthesis and therefore usual contraindications apply such as asthma, renal dysfunction, peptic ulceration and bleeding. In 2005 The European Medicines Agency (EMA) review on cox-2 specific inhibitors such as rofecoxib and paracoxib identified an increased risk of thrombotic events such as myocardial infarction and stroke. This has led to an increased reluctance to use cox-2 inhibitors intra-operatively. However the pectus population are young and fit and so advantages outweigh the risks in these patients. Indeed cox-2 inhibitors may have advantages in patients at risk of increased bleeding and gastric ulceration (PROSPECT Website).

Paracetamol

Paracetamol is also a useful adjunct to an opiate-based technique. The mechanism of action of paracetamol has not been entirely elucidated but there is evidence that it also works on cox-2 receptors, predominantly in the central nervous system. Intravenous paracetamol is highly effective as it has 100 % bio-availability avoiding first pass metabolism in the liver in comparison with oral or rectal preparations. It can be given in conjunction with NSAIDs. One gram of intravenous paracetamol is said to have similar analgesic efficacy to 10 mg of Intra-muscular morphine [5].

Other Novel Agents

Other more novel analgesics can be used intra-operatively or in the recovery room in patients with refractory pain.

Ketamine

Ketamine is an N methyl D aspartate (NMDA) receptor antagonist which has profound anaesthetic and analgesic properties, in small doses administered either intra-venously or intra-muscularly. It is opiate-sparing, reducing opiate side-effects such as respiratory depression. It may also prevent spinal-sensitisation or 'wind-up' which is attributed to the development of chronic post-operative pain syndromes. Intramuscular administration has some advantages in that the effects of the ketamine are more prolonged. It can also be given as an infusion in the post-operative period.

Clonidine

Clonidine is an alpha-2 adrenergic agonist and imidazoline receptor antagonist. It was originally used to treat hypertension, but has several off-licence uses which include sedation and the treatment of pain. It can be used in conjunction with opiates intra-operatively and in the recovery room and can also be given as an infusion. It works by an entirely different mechanism from opiates and therefore has a synergistic effect.

Gabapentin or Pre-gabalin

Gabapentin or Pre-gabalin were originally developed as anti-epileptic medications, but are now used in the treatment of neuropathic pain. They have similar structures to the neurotransmitter GABA and bind to voltage-dependent calcium channels, but their mechanism of action is unclear. There is limited evidence from other areas of surgery that pre-operative gabapentin may confer advantages in the management of post-operative pain. They reduce opiate usages and decrease opiate side effects. They may also have a theoretical role in the prevention of the development of chronic post-operative pain [6]. There is currently no published evidence for their use in Nuss surgery.

Wound Infiltration with Local Anaesthetic

Local wound infiltration by the surgeon at the time of surgery is a useful, simple and safe adjunct in the management of post-operative pain. Longer-acting local anaesthetics such as bupivacaine or ropivacaine should be used and the inclusion of adrenaline can prolong the duration of action further.

Paravertebral Nerve Blocks and Intercostal Nerve Blocks

Paravertebral blocks have been suggested as an alternative to thoracic epidural analgesia and a small study comparing bilateral paravertebral blocks with thoracic epidurals was published in 2014. Paravertebral blocks are technically easier to perform and have less serious complications than central neuraxial blockade. They can be performed as a 'one-shot' technique, by the anaesthetist prior to surgery or indwelling paravertebral catheters placed for use with infusions of local anaesthetic in the post-operative period. The major risk with bilateral paravertebral blockade is bilateral pneumothoraces. Ultrasound-guidance for block placement may reduce this risk. A retrospective study comparing 10 thoracic epidurals with 10 bilateral para-vertebral blocks in 20 adolescent males undergoing the Nuss procedure, showed no difference in post-operative opiate consumption or pain scores between the two groups [7].

Two meta-analyses and systemic reviews comparing epidural analagesia with paravertebral blockade in thoracotomy patients, concluded that analgesic efficacy was similar. However the side effect profile, including urinary retention, nausea and vomiting and pulmonary complications were lower in the paravertebral group [8, 9].

Similarly bilateral intercostal blocks performed prior to surgery by the anaesthetist or during surgery by the surgeon may be an alternative to central neuraxial blockade [10]. A recent double-blind randomized controlled trial comparing single-shot intercostal blocks performed with levobupivicaine or saline in 60 patients, showed decreased morphine consumption at surgery and for the first 6 h post-operatively, with less nausea and vomiting and less urinary retention in the levobupiviaine group [11].

Thoracic Epidural Analgesia

Thoracic epidural analgesia has been considered to be the gold-standard in pain management in surgery for the correction of chest-wall deformities. Thoracic epidurals must be placed with the patients awake or only mildly sedated to minimise the risk of neurological complications. This is a challenge in the paediatric or adolescent population and requires a co-operative patient and a skilled operator. Epidural analgesia has major side-effects and sequelae including intra-operative and post-operative hypotension, urinary retention, delayed mobilisation, inadequate analgesia, missed segments and patchy block. Epidural haematoma or abscess and spinal cord ischemia are major life-changing sequalae that require prompt detection and immediate neurosurgical imaging and intervention. This is not always rapidly available in cardiothoracic centres. Epidurals require assiduous nursing care and observations and have to be nursed on high-dependency units in many hospitals. This has cost and man-power implications.

There is also controversy about thromboprophylaxis with an epidural catheter in situ. Timing of low-molecular heparin administration must be co-ordinated with epidural placement and catheter removal. Heparin should not be given until 6 h post catheter insertion. Catheter removal must take place at trough levels of low molecular weight heparin and the subsequent dose should not be given until 6 h after catheter removal, to minimise the risk of epidural haematoma [12].

NAP3 (National Audi Project 3) carried out by the Royal College of Anaesthetists in the UK and published in January 2009 showed a major complication rate of 4.2 in 10,0000 central neuraxial blocks including spinals, epidurals and combine spinal-epidural techniques. This was a large study carried out over a 12 month period in the UK which included 70,0000 procedures. These broke down into 46 % spinals and 41 % epidurals. Forty-five percent of the epidurals were performed in obstetrics and 44 % for perioperative analgesia. There were 30 permanent injuries of which 60 % were in patients with epidurals. Eighty percent of the permanent epidural injuries were in the peri-operative group. Although complications rates were low, they occurred predominantly with peri-operative epidurals and the prognosis for vertebral canal haematoma or spinal cord ischaemia is extremely poor [13]. This may have discouraged the use of epidural analgesia in major surgery in the UK. The lack of convincing evidence that epidural anaesthesia decreases morbidity and improves patient outcome has also lead to anaesthetists re-evaluating whether the risks of epidural catheter placement, justify the benefits of the procedure [14].

Further to this, the National Pneumonectomy Study was published in the Journal of Cardiothoracic Surgery in 2009. This looked at 312 pneumonectomies for lung cancer over a 12 month period performed in 28 thoracic surgical centres in the UK. Major complications included significant arrhythmias requiring treatment (19.9 %), unexpected ICU admissions (9.3 %), 30 day mortality (5.4 %), further surgery (4.8 %) and increased inotrope usage (3.5 %). Sixty-one percent of the patients had a thoracic epidural and 31 % a paravertebral block. Risk factors for major complications included epidural analgesia, pre-operative ASA status, age and pre-operative lung function (DLCO, Diffusion capacity of the lung for carbon monoxide). This may be explained by increased hypotension and increased pulmonary complications with epidurals as opposed to a unilateral paravertebral block [15].

However, despite the published studies and audits, epidural analgesia remains the mainstay of perioperative pain management for pectus surgery in European and North American centres. A large multi-centre survey published in the Scandinavian literature in 2014 reported 91 % of institutions used epidurals for primary pain management [2]. Other studies have shown epidurals to provide superior analgesia to PCA Opiates in the immediate postoperative period, with moderately lower pain scores up to 48 h post-operatively [3]. A randomised study of epidural versus patient controlled analgesia was published in 2012 and included 110 patients. Epidurals were failed to be placed or did not work in 22 % of patients and epidural insertion significantly prolonged operative time. It also demonstrated marginally improved pain scores in the epidural group, but also greater demands on hospital staff with more calls to anaesthesia. There was no difference in hospital stay between the two groups [16]. The assumption that epidural analgesia is the truly the best pain management strategy for Nuss surgery is therefore being questioned. Patients who do not have epidurals have a shorter operating room time, less urinary retention and catheterisation, a shorter transition to oral medication and shorter hospitalisation [17].

Thoracic Epidural Analgesia is certainly a good option in centres with experienced epiduralists, nursing staff and facilities that can successfully monitor and manage epidural infusions and complications on the wards, with the availability of 24 h neuro-imaging and neurosurgery to manage catastrophic complications. If this is not available there should be some reluctance to place epidural catheters in young fit patients, who do not have cancer and are undergoing surgery primarily for aesthetic and psychological reasons.

Lumbar Spinal Opiates

Lumbar spinal opiates are another potential method of pain relief for Nuss surgery. Spinal diamorphine or preservative-free morphine is used extensively in enhanced recovery protocols for other types of surgery including major gynaecology, colorectal and orthopaedic surgery.

A large meta-analysis of intrathecal morphine in cardiac, thoracic, abdominal and spinal surgery showed opioid requirements were decreased intra-operatively and up to 48 h post-operatively [18]. There is no data for the use of spinal morphine or diamorphine in pectus surgery.

Hypnosis

They have been reports that post-operative self-hypnosis can improve pain scores, decrease opiate usage and decrease hospital stay [19].

A multi-modal approach to post-operative analgesia using a combination of neuraxial blockade or peripheral nerve block and pharmacological agents is probably the most successful strategy. This reduces the total dose of a single agent (i.e. opiate sparing), therefore minimising side-effects. Different classes of analgesics work by different mechanisms on different receptors and therefore have a synergistic effect when used in combination.

Step-Down Analgesia

When the epidural or PCA is discontinued, multi-modal regular analgesia should be prescribed. A combination of a non-steroidal anti-inflammatory drug, paracetamol and an oral opiate such as oromorph, is appropriate. The patient should be supplied with a similar combination of medication on discharge from hospital. The strong opiate can be replaced by a weak opiate such as codeine or tramadol.

Post-operative Care

Of equal importance to the post-operative analgesic technique is the ward environment, standards of observation, monitoring, and nursing care. Patients with epidural infusions need cardiovascular, neurological and respiratory observations to detect rising epidural block, respiratory compromise, hypotension and neurological complications. This requires nursing staff to be trained in the management of epidurals. This level of care can only be provided in a high dependency or intensive care environment in many institutions.

Patients with opiate patient controlled analgesia also need regular respiratory observations (respiratory rate and depth) and assessment of level of sedation. This should be achievable in a surgical ward environment. The analgesic technique therefore has implications for the acuity of post-operative care and high-dependency bed utilisation.

Chronic Pain Management

There is no published data on the incidence of chronic pain after the Nuss procedure. However we know that 67 % of patients develop chronic pain after thoracotomy, which persists in 25 % of cases [20]. Risk factors for the development of chronic pain included longer and more complicated surgical procedures and severe post-operative pain [21]. This provides further impetus to achieve excellent pain control in the perioperative period. This patient group also needs access to anaesthetists trained in chronic pain management and a multi-disciplinary chronic pain service, in the event of the development of post-operative chronic pain syndromes.

References

1. Castellani C, Schalamon J, Saxena AK, Hoellwarth ME. Early complications of the Nuss procedure for pectus excavatum a prospective study. Pediatr Surg Int. 2008;24(6):659–66.
2. Muhly WT, Maxwell LG, Cravero JP. Pain management following the Nuss procedure: a survey of practice and review. Acta Anaesthesiol Scand. 2014;58(9): 1134–9.
3. Stroud AM, Tulanont DD, Goates TE, Goodnev PP, Croitoru D. Epidural analgesia versus intravenous patient-controlled analgesia following minimally invasive pectus excavatum repair: a systemic review and meta-analysis. J Pediatr Surg. 2014;9(5):798–806.
4. Grosen K, Pfeiffer-Jensen M, Pilegaard HK. Postoperative consumption of opioid analgesics following correction of pectus excavatum is influenced by pectus severity: a single-centre study of 236 patients undergoing minimally invasive correction of pectus excavatum. Eur J Cardiothorac Surg. 2010;37(4):833–9.

5. Van Aken H, Thys L, Veekman L, Buerkle H. Assessing analgesia in a single and repeated adminis-trations or propacetamol for postoperative pain: com-parison with morphine after dental surgery. Anesth Analg. 2004;98:159–65.

6. Clarke H, Bonin RP, Orser BA, Englesaki M, Wijeysundera DN, Katz J. The prevention of chronic postsurgical pain using gabapentin and pre-gabalin: a combined systemic review and meta-analysis. Anesth Analg. 2012;115(2):428–42.

7. Hall Burton DM, Boretsky KR. A comparison of para-vertebral nerve block catheters and thoracic epidural catheters for post-operative analgesia following the Nuss procedure for pectus excavatum repair. Paediatr Anaesth. 2014;24(5):516–20.

8. Davies RG, Myles PS, Graham JM. A comparison of the analgesic efficacy and side-effects of paravertebral vs epidural blockade for thoracotomy – a systematic review and meta-analysis of randomized trials. Br J Anaesth. 2006;96:418–42.

9. Joshi GP, Bonnet F, Shah R, Wilkinson RC, Camu F, Fischer B, Neugebauer EA, Rawal N, Schug SA, Simanski C, Kehlet H. A systematic review of random-ized trials evaluating regional techniques for postthora-cotomy analgesia. Anesth Analg. 2008;107:1026–40.

10. Lukošienė L, Kalibatienė L, Barauskas V. Intercostal nerve block in pediatric minimally invasive thoracic surgery. Acta Medica Lituanica. 2012;19(3):150.

11. Lukosiene L, Macas A, Trepenaltis D, Malcius D, Barauskas V. Single shot intercostal block for pain management in pediatric patients undergoing the Nuss procedure: a double blind randomised con-trolled study. J Pediatr Surg. 2014;49 (12):1735–7.

12. Horlocker TT. Regional anaesthesia in a patient receiving antithrombotic and anti-patelet therapy. Br J of Anaesth. 2011;107(S1):96–106.

13. NAP3 Report and findings of the third National Audit Project of the Royal College of Anaesthetists. Pages 1–36. Published by the Royal College of Anaesthetists; 2009.

14. Wildsmith JA. Continuous thoracic epidural block for surgery: gold standard or debased currency? Br J Anaesth. 2012;109(1):9–12.

15. Powell ES, Pearce AC, Cook D, Davies P, Bishay E, Bowler GM, Gao F, UKPOS Co-ordinators. UK pneu-monectomy outcome study (UKPOS): a prospective observational study of pneumonectomy outcome. J Cardiothorac Surg. 2009;30:4–41.

16. St Peter SD, Weesner KA, Weissend EE, Sharp SW, Valusek PA, Sharp RJ, Snyder CL, Hotcomb 3rd GW, Ostlie DJ. Epidural vs patient-controlled analgesia for postoperative pain after pectus excavatum repair: a prospective randomized trial. J Pediatr Surg. 2012; 47(1):148–53.

17. St Peter SD, Weesner KA, Sharp RJ, Sharp SW, Ostlie DJ, Hotcomb 3rd GW. Is epidural analgesia truly the best pain management strategy after minimally invasive pectus excavatum repair? J Pediatr Surg. 2008;43(1):79–82.

18. Meylan N, Elia N, Lysakowski C, Tramer MR. Benefit and risk of intrathecal morphine without local anaesthetic in patients undergoing major surgery: meta-analysis of randomized trials. Br J Anaesth. 2009;102(2):156–67.

19. Lobe TE. Perioperative hypnosis reduces hospitalisa-tion in patients undergoing the Nuss procedure excavatum. J Laparoendosc Adv Surg Tech A. 2006; 16(6):639–42.

20. Perttunen K, Tasmuth T, Kalso E. Chronic pain after thoracic surgery: a follow up study. Acta Anaesthesiol Scand. 1999;43(5):563–7.

21. Katz J, Jackson M, Kavanagh BP, Sandler AN. Acute pain after thoracic surgery predicts long-term post-thoracotomy pain. Clin J Pain. 1996;12(1):50–5.

Cardiopulmonary Function in Relation to Pectus Excavatum

12

Marie Maagaard and Hans K. Pilegaard

Abstract

Pectus excavatum (PE) is the most common, congenital deformity of the anterior chest wall and represents around 90 % of all anomalies of the anterior chest wall. PE has been very well investigated over the years with a vast amount of studies being produced, still, no consensus has yet been reached on the direct impact of PE on cardiopulmonary function.

Keywords

Cardiopulmonary function • Pectus Excavatum • Chest wall deformity • Congenital deformity • Anterior chest wall

Pectus excavatum (PE) is the most common, congenital deformity of the anterior chest wall and represents around 90 % of all anomalies of the anterior chest wall. PE has been very well investigated over the years with a vast amount of studies being produced, still, no consensus has yet

M. Maagaard, PhD Student
Department of Cardiothoracic and Vascular Surgery, Department of Clinical Medicine, Aarhus University Hospital, Denmark, Aarhus, Denmark

Department of Clinical Medicine,
Aarhus University Hospital, Aarhus, Denmark

H.K. Pilegaard, MD (✉)
Associate Professor, Department of Cardiothoracic and Vascular Surgery, Department of Clinical Medicine, Aarhus University Hospital, Denmark, Aarhus, Denmark
e-mail: pilegaard@dadlnet.dk

been reached on the direct impact of PE on cardiopulmonary function.

The question of a possible impact on cardiopulmonary function was raised as early as in the 1920s, where the German thoracic surgeon Dr Sauerbruch [1], reported on a young adult who was suffering from PE and complained about increasing dyspnoea and being exhausted easily. The patient underwent surgery and some years following the surgery, he reported back with clear subjective improvements and was now able to work for hours a day without being exhausted as easily.

Many other cases like that of Dr Sauerbruch have since been presented, where patients preoperatively present with symptoms of varying degree, with more than 60 % presenting with exercise intolerance, lack of endurance and shortness of breath [2]. Through the last 20 years, after the minimal technique by dr. Nuss was introduced

[3]; a great amount of patients in their early teens have undergone corrective surgery with cosmetically great results, and therefore the question has never been more interesting than now. In several papers, where patients and parents describe the changes of the patients' lives following surgery, it is well-documented that it is not just the appearance that changes, but also their physical exercise capacity. Likewise, any preoperative symptoms that may have been described are reported as nearly disappeared or decreased following surgery. Accordingly, many studies have focused their investigation on this change happening with the patient undergoing surgery.

The psychosocial change reported following surgery has recently been examined thoroughly by a research group from our institution at Aarhus University hospital in Denmark [4]. With this study, Jacobsen et al. have published results on a large patient-group of 172 children who were all undergoing the minimally invasive Nuss procedure. They were asked about their health-related quality of life following corrective surgery for PE, and the same type of questionnaire was also handed out to a healthy control-group of 387 age-matched schoolchildren. All the participants were between the ages of 8–20 years. Uniquely for the patients, they were also asked to fill out the Nuss Assessment Questionnaire, which retrospectively investigated possible changes in perceived physical and psychosocial aspects following the Nuss operation.

The Nuss Assessment Questionnaire found the patients to report of an increased self-esteem and body-concept postoperatively. The other questionnaire, which looked at differences between the patient and the control group, found that the perceived health related quality of life was higher in the patients compared to controls. Furthermore, the patients even reported of a higher physical functioning compared to the controls. Other studies have found similar results. In North America, Kelly et al. published an article on patients reporting of markedly improved body image and perceived ability for physical activity following corrective surgery [5]. And as recent as October 2014, Kuru et al. [6] found comparable results with that of Jacobsen et al. In short, there can be no doubt of the positive impact that surgery has on most of the patients' body image and self-esteem.

In light of the abovementioned findings, the interesting subject is clearly whether these reported changes following surgery can be attributed solely to the changed body image and bettered self-esteem – or if the surgery also has a physiological impact on the patients' physical capacity? When considering studies based on resting cardiac function in patients suffering from PE, no noticeable impact on the cardiopulmonary function has yet been established [7]. But during exercise, different reports have noted a measurable, decreased stamina among patients [8, 9].

With a study from 2005, Rowland and colleagues [8] examined patients with PE preoperatively, and matched them with age-matched healthy controls. All participants were in their early teens and went through upright bicycle exercise tests. As an important detail, the authors also considered the habitual exercise levels of the participants by handing out questionnaires. The exercise tests showed a decreased cardiac index (cardiac output compared to the individual's body surface area) reached in the patient group during maximal exercise. This could not be attributed to a difference in habitual exercise level between the two groups. Similar results have been noted in other, small-scale studies. However, common for these pre-operative studies are that they lack follow-up testing after the funnel chest has been corrected.

A couple of studies have looked at the patients after follow-up and find there is a sustained significant increase in cardiac performance. Neviere et al. followed 70 adult patients, age 18–62 years, after correction by a modified Ravitch procedure for 12 months and found that the maximal O_2 uptake measured during exercise increased significantly from 77 ± 2 % to 87 ± 2 %, $p < 0.01$ [10]. Another group, O'Keefe and colleagues looked at cardiopulmonary exercise function in young adults following surgery after the Nuss procedure [11]. Sixty-seven patients at age 14 years were included prior to surgery. Through increased bicycle exercise testing, their exercise O_2-pulse (a surrogate for stroke volume during exercise) were measured and compared to post-operative measurements. Following bar-removal, O'Keefe noted a significant increase in O_2-pulse during exercise. They also investigated cardiac index before and after surgery, although without significant difference. It should be emphasized though that this parameter was measured at rest and the findings are thus in line with those of former studies.

Another important aspect that should be pointed out with this study by O'Keefe is that there is no comparable control group. Therefore it is impossible to judge whether the improved exercise function found is caused by the impact of surgery or simply by the concurrent growth of the patients. As noted earlier, they were circa 14 years of age at inclusion and on average 3 years older at the time of follow-up.

At our institution in Denmark, we set out to take all factors in to mind – including a comparable control group, investigated during exercise and tested both before and after surgery. The results after 3 years follow-up were published in 2013 [12]. The exercise capacity of teenagers was examined before undergoing the Nuss procedure and compared to a group of healthy, age-matched control subjects. Furthermore, the habitual exercise levels were documented through all 3 years. Prior to surgery, we found teenagers with PE to have a lower maximal cardiac index (CI_{max}) compared to a group of healthy age-matched controls during incremental bicycle exercise [13]. One year following the modified Nuss procedure patients had significantly increased their CI_{max} during exercise, however still scoring significantly lower compared to the age-matched controls [14].

The same study-population was investigated again after the pectus bar-removal in order to determine whether patients would further increase their cardiopulmonary function to a level comparable with the healthy, age-matched control subjects, and in this way continuously taking growth during the investigational period into consideration. Following the bar-removal the cardiac exercise parameters had increased in the patients to such a level, that no difference existed between the two groups anymore. In other words, the patient group had normalized their maximum cardiac index during exercise.

The exercise results from our 3-year follow-up study are illustrated in Fig. 12.1. When looking at the patient group, a significant increase of 21 % was found within this group over the 3 years – a similar increase could not be found in the control subjects. With these results it is thus emphasized that the change found in the patient group could not solely be attributed to the concurrent growth during the investigational period.

The maximum heart rate reached during the exercise tests did not differ between the two groups during the 3 years. And much like Rowland et al. we also considered the possible different habitual exercise habits of the patients and the control subjects. However, at no point during the 3 years did we find any significant difference between the groups. The increased exercise function could

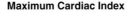

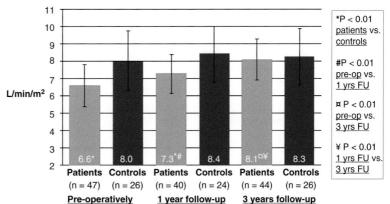

Fig. 12.1 Maximum cardiac index (With permission from Maagaard et al. [12])

thereby not be explained by a higher level of physical activity following the corrective surgery.

The Haller Index was also examined by MRI in both groups throughout the 3 years follow-up study and these measurements showed a significant decrease in the indices in the patient group, with no changes seen in the control group. No difference existed between the groups following bar-removal. But in contrast to the study done by Swanson et al. [15], we did not find any correlation between a decreased cardiac exercise function and a high Haller index. In other words, it was not the severity of the chest wall deformity in our study that determined the level of reduced exercise function.

Echocardiographic studies investigating postoperative results both after the Ravitch and also the Nuss Procedure have shown an increased right ventricular end-diastolic diameter, which might be caused by the decreased pressure from the sternum, causing better filling of the right ventricle. However, these studies are only done at rest [16, 17].

With these results it is illustrated that following corrective surgery, the cardiac exercise function of the patients with PE normalizes compared to a healthy, age-matched control group and also increases the cardiac performance in adults. Surgical correction of PE should be considered in all patients who presents with symptoms of reduced physical performance and not only for patients with cosmetic complaints.

References

1. Sauerbruch F. Die chirurgie die brustorgane. From Springer Forlag or Verlag von Julius Springer; 1920. p. 437–44.
2. Kelly Jr RE. Pectus excavatum: historical background, clinical picture, preoperative evaluation and criteria for operation. Semin Pediatr Surg. 2008;17:181–93.
3. Nuss D, Kelly Jr RE, Croitoru DP, Katz ME. A 10-year review of a minimally invasive technique for the correction of pectus excavatum. J Pediatr Surg. 1998;33:545–52.
4. Jacobsen EB, Thastum M, Jeppesen JH, Pilegaard HK. Health-related quality of life in children and adolescents undergoing surgery for pectus excavatum. Eur J Pediatr Surg. 2010;20:85–91.
5. Kelly RE, Cash TF, Shamberger RC, Mitchell KK, Mellins RB, Lawson ML, Oldham K, Azizkhan RG,

Hebra AV, Nuss D, Goretsky MJ, Sharp RJ, Holcomb GW, Shim WKT, Megison SM, Moss RL, Fecteau AH, Colombani PM, Bagley T, Quinn A, Moskowitz AB. Surgical repair of pectus excavatum markedly improves body image and perceived ability for physical activity: multicenter study. Pediatrics. 2008;122: 1218–22.
6. Kuru P, Bostanci K, Ermerak NO, Bahadir AT, Afacan C, Yuksel M. Quality of life improves after minimally invasive repair of pectus excavatum. Asian Cardiovasc Thorac Ann. 2015;23(3):302–7.
7. Beiser GD, Epstein SE, Stampfer M, Goldstein RE, Noland SP, Levitsky S. Impairment of cardiac function in patients with pectus excavatum, with improvement after operative correction. N Engl J Med. 1972;287:267–72.
8. Rowland T, Moriarty K, Banever G. Effect of pectus excavatum deformity on cardiorespiratory fitness in adolescent boys. Arch Pediatr Adolesc Med. 2005; 159:1069–73.
9. Malek MH, Fonkalsrud EW, Cooper CB. Ventilatory and cardiovascular responses to exercise in patients with pectus excavatum. Chest. 2003;124:870–82.
10. Neviere R, Montaigne D, Benhamed L, Catto M, Edme JL, Matran R, Wurtz A. Cardiopulmonary response following surgical repair of pectus excavatum in adult patients. Eur J Cardiothorac Surg. 2011; 40:e77–82.
11. O'Keefe J, Byrne R, Montgomery M, Harder J, Roberts D, Sigalet DL. Longer term effects of closed repair of pectus excavatum on cardiopulmonary status. J Pediatr Surg. 2013;48:1049–54.
12. Maagaard M, Tang M, Ringgaard S, Nielsen HH, Frokiaer J, Haubuf M, Pilegaard HK, Hjortdal VE. Normalized cardiopulmonary exercise function in patients with pectus excavatum three years after operation. Ann Thorac Surg. 2013;96(1):272–8.
13. Lesbo M, Tang M, Nielsen HHM, Frøkiær J, Lundorf E, Pilegaard HK, Hjortdal VE. Compromised cardiac function in exercising teenagers with pectus excavatum. Interact Cardiovasc Thorac Surg. 2011;13:377–80.
14. Tang M, Nielsen HHM, Lesbo M, Frokiaer J, Maagaard M, Pilegaard HK, Hjortdal VE. Improved cardiopulmonary exercise function after modified Nuss operation for pectus excavatum. Eur J Cardiothorac Surg. 2012;41:1063–7.
15. Swanson JW, Avansino JR, Phillips GS, Yung D, Whitlock KB, Redding GJ, Sawin RS. Correlating Haller Index and cardiopulmonary disease in pectus excavatum. Am J Surg. 2012;203:660–4.
16. Krueger T, Chassot PG, Christodoulou M, Cheng C, Ris HB, Magnusson L. Cardiac function assessed by transesophageal echocardiography during pectus excavatum repair. Ann Thorac Surg. 2010;89:240–3.
17. Gurkan U, Aydemir B, Aksoy S, Akgoz H, Tosu AR, Oz D, Gungor B, Yilmaz H, Bolca O. Echocardiographic assessment of right ventricular function before and after surgery in patients with pectus excavatum and right ventricular compression. Thorac Cardiovasc Surg. 2014;62:231–5.

Other Chest Wall Deformities

13

Shyam K. Kolvekar and Nikolaos Panagiotopoulos

Abstract

There are various other chest wall deformities that are worth discussing. These will be outlined in the following chapter. Jeune Syndrome, also known as Asphyxiating Thoracic Dystrophy (ATD) is a rare autosomal recessive skeletal dysplasia with multiorgan involvement. It was first described by Jeune in 1954 and it affects 1 per 10,0000–13,0000 live births. There are two subtypes of the syndrome with severe subtype being incompatible with life. Poland syndrome (PS) is classified as a chondro-costal chest wall deformity with main clinical manifestation the underdevelopment or absence of the major pectorals muscle. It is a congenital unilateral chest wall deformity that affects both males and females in a ratio of 3:1 and with an incident variation from 1–7,0000 to 1–10,0000 live births. A rarer category of chest wall deformation is pectus arcuatum represents a rare category of chest wall deformities in the family of pectus anomalies and It includes mixed excavatum and carinatum features along a longitudinal or transversal axis resulting in a multiplanar curvature of the sternum and adjacent ribs. Sternal cleft represents a rare idiopathic chest wall deformity caused by a defect in the sternum's fusion process. It accounts for 0.15 % of all chest wall deformities and there is an association with the Hexb gene. There are four types of sternal clefts according to the classification proposed by Schamberger and Welch in 1990.

S.K. Kolvekar, MS, MCh, FRCS, FRCSCTh (✉)
Department of Cardiothoracic Surgery,
University College London Hospitals,
The Heart Hospital & Barts Heart Center, London, UK
e-mail: kolvekar@yahoo.com

N. Panagiotopoulos, MD, PhD
Department of Cardiothoracic Surgery,
University College London Hospitals (UCLH),
London, UK

© Springer International Publishing Switzerland 2016
S.K. Kolvekar, H.K. Pilegaard (eds.), *Chest Wall Deformities and Corrective Procedures*,
DOI 10.1007/978-3-319-23968-2_13

Keywords
Poland syndrome • Jeune Syndrome • Asphyxiating Thoracic Dystrophy
• Congenital chest wall deformity • Pectus Arcuatum • Sternal cleft
• Sternum's fusion process

Jeune Syndrome

Jeune Syndrome, also known as Asphyxiating Thoracic Dystrophy (ATD) is a rare autosomal recessive skeletal dysplasia with multiorgan involvement. It was first described by Jeune [1] in 1954 in a pair of siblings and it affects 1 per 10,0000–13,0000 live births [2]. The inheritance of ATD is autosomal recessive. A genetic locus has been identified on chromosome 15q13 as well in the IFT8o gene encoding an intraflagellar protein in a subset of patients with no extraskeletal manifestations [3]. Mainly there are two subtypes of the syndrome:

- Severe type: Accounts for 70 % of cases and usually is lethal in infancy. It is associated with extremely small thorax and respiratory failure is the rule.
- Mild type: Found in 30 % of cases and is correlated with better prognosis and prolonged survival. Renal or liver dysfunction can be present.

Clinically the Jeune syndrome is associated with respiratory failure secondary to reduced Anteroposterior and lateral diameters of the thorax [3–7]. Radiographically the chest is narrow – bell shaped with short horizontal ribs and elevated clavicles. Additional coexisting bone anomalies include sort limbs and small irregular pelvis and postaxial polydactyly of both hands and feet [8–14]. Prenatal diagnosis can be established with ultrasound as early as 14 weeks (Fig. 13.1) [16–18].

Poland Syndrome

Poland syndrome (PS) is classified as a chondrocostal chest wall deformity with main clinical manifestation the underdevelopment or absence of the major pectorals muscle (Fig. 13.2). It was Alfred Poland a British surgeon at Guys Hospital in 1840 that reported the partial absence of major pectoralis muscle in cadavers and ipsilateral deformity of the hand in the same cadaver but without associating these two anomalies [19]. Crarkson a plastic and hand surgeon almost 100 years later in 1962 and in the same hospital reported the association of these two anomalies and gave Poland s syndrome identity [20]. The etiology still remains unknown and only few theories have been reported in the literature. The most accredited hypothesis is the interruption of the vascular supply in subclavian and vertebral artery during embryonic life that leads to different malformations [21]. Another theory includes paradominant inheritance or the presence of a lethal gene survival by mosaicism [22]. Poland syndrome is a congenital unilateral chest wall deformity that affects both males and females with aeration of 3:1 and with an incident variation from 1–7,0000 to 1–10,0000 live births [23]. Patients with PS are usually a symptomatic and there is no limitation due to muscle defects. Key features for the diagnosis of Poland syndrome include partial or complete absence of the pectoralis major muscle and associated breast deformity. The breast anomaly ranges from mild asymmetry of shape and size including the nipple complex to severe hypoplasia or aphasia including atheling or polythelia. Upper limb is usually involved from the classical symbrachydactily to split hand or other defects [24, 25]. Cardiac and renal anomalies have also been reported as well as dextroposition [26] and scoliosis [27]. Finally other chest wall deformities can co-exist with pectus excavatum and pectus carinatum.

Pectus Arcuatum

Pectus arcuatum represents a rare category of chest wall deformities in the family of pectus anomalies and is derived from the latin word

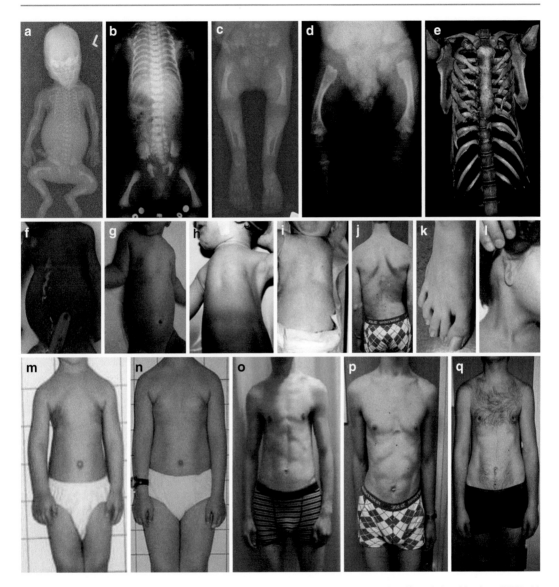

Fig. 13.1 Clinical features of *DYNC2H1* patients. (**a–e**) Hallmarks of Jeune asphyxiating thoracic dystrophy (JATD): (**a**, JATD-5; **b**, JATD-16) Small thorax due to short ribs; (**a**, JATD-5, **b**, JATD-16, **c**, JATD-5, **d**, JATD-14) Small ilia with acetabular spurs; (**c**, JATD-5, **d**, JATD-14) Shortening of femurs, accompanied by bowing in (**d**, JATD-14); (**e**) 3D reconstruction of CT images of patient JATD-4. (**f–i**) Severity of the rib shortening varies between different patients from different families carrying *DYNC2H1* mutations as well as between affected siblings: while patient JATD-5 presents with extremely shortened ribs (**f**), patient JATD-18 (UCL62.2) is only mildly affected (**g**). (**h, i**) Patient JATD-14 (**h**, UCL80.1) is markably more severely affected than his sister JATD-14 (**i**, UCL80.2). (**j–l**) Additional features: (**j**) scoliosis in JATD-2, (**k**) syndactyly in JATD-2, (**l**) ear malformation in JATD-16. (**m–q**) Thoracic narrowing becomes less pronounced with increasing patient age. (**m**) Shows patient JATD-16 at under 5 years; the same patient is shown a few years later in (**n**) at under 10 years. (**o**) Patient JATD-3 in his 20s, (**p**) patient JATD-2 in his late teens, (**q**) patient JATD-1 in his mid-20s these cases have less pronounced thoracic phenotypes compared to birth or infancy, as described in the text. Note also that shortening of the upper limbs seems less severe when JATD patients reach adolescence (With permission from Schmidts et al. [15])

Poland's Syndrome   **Pectus Arcuatum or Pouter Pigeon Breast**

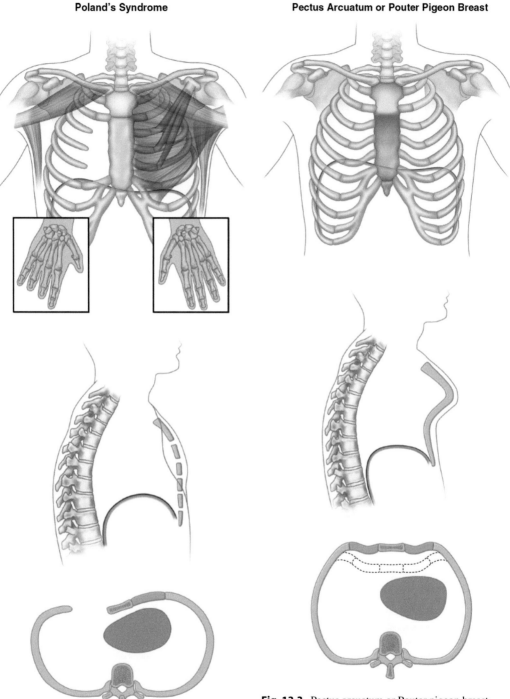

Fig. 13.3 Pectus arcuatum or Pouter pigeon breast

Fig. 13.2 Poland's syndrome

arcus meaning an arch or curvature (Fig. 13.3). It includes mixed excavatum and carinatum features along a longitudinal or transversal axis resulting in a multiplanar curvature of the sternum and adjacent ribs [28]. This clinical condition usually coexists with Poland syndrome and it has been correlated with cardiac abnormalities such as ventricular septum defect [29].

Sternal Anomalies – Sternal Cleft

Sternal cleft represents a rare idiopathic chest wall deformity caused by a defect in the sternum's fusion process (Fig. 13.4). It accounts for 0.15 % of all chest wall deformities [30] and there is an a association with the Hexb gene [31]. According to the classification proposed by Schamberger and Welch in 1990 there are four types of sternal clefts [32]:

- Thoracic ectopic cordis. The heart is ectopic and not covered by skin. The chest cavity is hypo plastic and is associated with very poor prognosis and with only few survivals following surgical intervention [33].
- Cervical ectopia cordis. More rare case than the above mentioned. The heart is more cranial, sometimes with the apex fused with the mouth. Prognosis is always negative.
- Thoracoabdominal ectopia cordis. The heart is covered by a thin membranous layer and is associated with an inferior sternal defect. It usually presents as part of pentalogy of Cantrell [34] and the prognosis after repair can be good.
- Sternum cleft- bifid sternum. It can be partial or complete as a result of deficiency in the midline embryonic fusion of the sternal valves [35].

Sternal clefts can be classified as complete, superior or inferior. Superior clefts can be U shaped if proximal to the fourth cartilage or V shaped if reaches the xiphoid process (Fig. 13.5). Before planning a surgical intervention other defects should be identified [36] and ruled out such as cardiac, aortic coarctation, eye abnormalities, hemangiomas, cleft lip or palate and gastroschisis.

Cleft Sternum

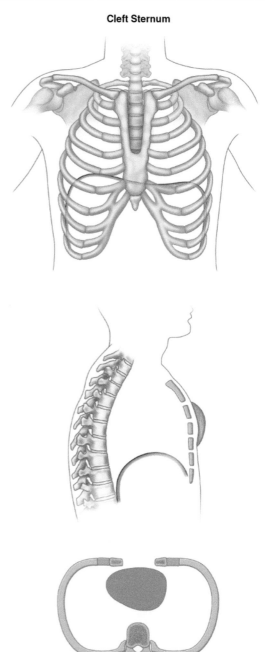

Fig. 13.4 Cleft sternum

Classification of sternal clefts

I. Main types

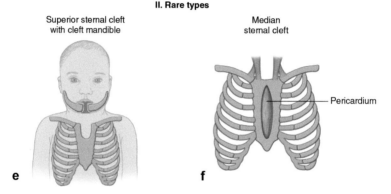

II. Rare types

Fig. 13.5 Classification of sternal clefts. *I* Main types. (**a**) Superior sternal cleft. (**b**) Subtotal sternal cleft. (**c**) Total sternal cleft. (**d**) Inferior sternal cleft. *II* Rare types. (**e**) Superior sternal cleft with cleft mandible. (**f**) Median sternal cleft

References

1. Jeune M, Carron R, Beraud C, Loaec Y. Polychondrodystrophie avec blocage thoracique d'évolution fatale. Pediatrie. 1954;9(4):390–2.
2. Oberklaid F, Danks DM, Mayne V, Campbell P. Asphyxiating thoracic dysplasia. Clinical, radiological, and pathological information on 10 patients. Arch Dis Child. 1977;52(10):758–65.
3. Beales PL, Bland E, Tobin JL, Bacchelli C, Tuysuz B, Hill J, Rix S, Pearson CG, Kai M, Hartley J, Johnson C, Irving M, Elcioglu N, Winey M, Tada M, Scambler PJ. IFT80, which encodes a conserved intraflagellar transport protein, is mutated in Jeune asphyxiating thoracic dystrophy. Nat Genet. 2007;39(6):727–9.
4. Amirou M, Bourdat-Michel G, Pinel N, Huet G, Gaultier J, Cochat P. Successful renal transplantation in Jeune syndrome type 2. Pediatr Nephrol. 1998;12(4):293–4.
5. Morgan NV, Bacchelli C, Gissen P, et al. A locus for asphyxiating thoracic dystrophy, ATD maps to chromosome 15q13. J Med Genet. 2003;40:431–5. doi:10.1136/jmg.40.6.431.
6. Oberklaid F, Danks DM, Mayne V, Campbell P. Asphyxiating thoracic dysplasia: clinical, radiological, and pathological information on 10 patients. Arch Dis Child. 1977;52:758–65. doi:10.1136/adc.52.10.758.
7. O'Connor MB, Gallagher DP, Mulloy E. Jeune syndrome. Postgrad Med J. 2008;84:559.
8. Barnes ND, Hull D, Simons JS. Thoracic dystrophy. Arch Dis Child. 1969;44:11–7.
9. Cortina H, Beltran J, Olague R, et al. The wide spectrum of the asphyxiating thoracic dysplasia. Pediatr Radiol. 1979;8:93–9.
10. Friedman JM, Kaplan HG, Hall JG. The Jeune syndrome (asphyxiating thoracic dystrophy) in an adult. Am J Med. 1975;59:857–62.
11. Hennekam RCM, Beemer FM, Gerards LJ, Cats B. Thoracic pelvic phalangeal dystrophy (Jeune syndrome). Tijdschr Kindergeneeskd. 1983;51:95–100.
12. Herdman RC, Langer LO. The thoracic asphyxiant dystrophy and renal disease. Am J Dis Child. 1968;116:192–201.
13. Kajantie E, Andersson S, Kaitila I. Familial asphyxiating thoracic dysplasia: clinical variability and impact of improved neonatal intensive care. J Pediatr. 2001;139:130–3.

14. Pirnar T, Neuhauser EBD. Asphyxiating thoracic dystrophy of the newborn. Am J Roentgenol Radium Ther Nucl Med. 1966;98:358–64.
15. Schmidts M, Arts HH, Bongers EM, et al. Exome sequencing identifies DYNC2H1 mutations as a common cause of asphyxiating thoracic dystrophy (Jeune syndrome) without major polydactyly, renal or retinal involvement. J Med Genet. 2013;50(5):309–23.
16. Chen CP, Lin SP, Liu FF, et al. Prenatal diagnosis of asphyxiating thoracic dysplasia (Jeune syndrome). Am J Perinatol. 1996;13:495–8.
17. den Hollander NS, Robben SGF, Hoogeboom AJM, et al. Early prenatal sonographic diagnosis and follow-up of Jeune syndrome. Ultrasound Obstet Gynecol. 2001;18:378–83.
18. Zimmer EZ, Weinraub Z, Raijman A, et al. Antenatal diagnosis of a fetus with an extremely narrow thorax and short limb dwarfism. J Clin Ultrasound. 1984;12:112–4.
19. Poland A. Deficiency of the pectoral muscles. Guys Hosp Rep. 1841;VI:191–3.
20. Clarkson P. Poland's syndactyly. Guys Hosp Rep. 1962;111:335–46.
21. Poullin P, Toussirot E, Schiano A, Serratrice G. Complete and dissociated forms of Poland's syndrome (5 cases). Rev Rhum Mal Osteoartic. 1992;59(2):114–20.
22. van Steensel MA. Poland anomaly: not unilateral or bilateral but mosaic. Am J Med Genet. 2004;125A(2):211–2.
23. Fokin A, Robicsek F. Poland's syndrome revisited. Ann Thorac Surg. 2002;74(6):2218.
24. Al-Qattan MM. Classification of hand anomalies in Poland's syndrome. Br J Plast Surg. 2001;54(2):132–6.
25. Shamberger RC, Welch KJ, Upton III J. Surgical treatment of thoracic deformity in Poland's syndrome. J Pediatr Surg. 1989;24(8):760–5.
26. Torre M, Baban A, Buluggiu A, Costanzo S, Bricco L, Lerone M, Bianca S, Gatti GL, Sénès FM, Valle M, Calevo MG. Dextrocardia in patients with Poland syndrome: phenotypic characterization provides insight into the pathogenesis. J Thorac Cardiovasc Surg. 2010;139(5):1177–82.
27. Alexander A, Fokin MD, Robicsek F. Poland's syndrome revisited. Ann Thorac Surg. 2002;74(6):2218–25.
28. Duhamel P, Brunel C, Le Pimpec F, Pons F, Jancovici R. Correction of the congenital malformations of the front chest by the modelling technique of sternochondroplasty: technique and results on a series of 14 cases. Ann Chir Plast Esthet. 2003;48:77–85.
29. Fokin AA. Pouter pigeon breast. Chest Surg Clin N Am. 2000;10:377–91.
30. Acastello E, Majluf F, Garrido P, Barbosa LM, Peredo A. Sternal cleft: a surgical opportunity. J Pediatr Surg. 2003;38(2):178–83.
31. Forzano F, Daubeney PE, White SM. Midline raphe, sternal cleft, and other midline abnormalities: a new dominant syndrome? Am J Med Genet A. 2005;135(1):9–12.
32. Shamberger R, Welch K. Sternal defects. Pediatr Surg Int. 1990;5:156–64.
33. Dobell AR, Williams HB, Long RW. Staged repair of ectopia cordis. J Pediatr Surg. 1982;17(4):353–8.
34. Cantrell JR, Haller JA, Ravitch MM. A syndrome of congenital defects involving the abdominal wall, sternum, diaphragm, pericardium, and heart. Surg Gynecol Obstet. 1958;107(5):602–14.
35. Acastello E. Patologias de la pared toracica en pediatria. Buenos Aires: Editorial El Ateneo; 2006.
36. Torre M, Rapuzzi G, Carlucci M, Pio L, Jasonni V. Phenotypic spectrum and management of sternal cleft: literature review and presentation of a new series. Eur J Cardiothorac Surg. 2012;41(1):4–9. doi:10.1016/j.ejcts.2011.05.049.

Acquired Chest Wall Deformities and Corrections

14

Herbert J. Witzke, Natalie L. Simon,
and Shyam K. Kolvekar

Abstract

Acquired deformities of the chest wall are malformations, which develop due to non-congenital causative factors. Based on etiology, three major categories of acquired chest wall malformations can be distinguished. (1) Primary disease of the chest wall itself can cause deformation of the chest wall. This includes tumors and infections affecting the chest wall with subsequent development of chest wall deformation. (2) The largest group of acquired chest wall deformities are iatrogenic in nature and occur as a result of previous surgical intervention to the chest wall, seen as acquired restrictive thoracic dystrophy or acquired Jeune's syndrome in young patients following open correction of pectus excavatum deformity. Iatrogenic chest wall deformities may also develop following rip graft harvesting or failed closure of thoracotomies. (3) Post-traumatic deformities are a result of direct or indirect trauma to the torso. This chapter is aimed to provide a comprehensive overview of the spectrum of acquired chest wall deformities and to discuss their pathophysiology, diagnosis and treatment.

Keywords

Acquired chest wall deformities • Iatrogenic • Post-traumatic • Acquired restrictive thoracic dystrophy • Acquired Jeune's syndrome • Acquired pectus carinatum • Chest wall tumor • Chest wall infection • Lung herniation

H.J. Witzke, MD
Department of Cardiothoracic Surgery,
University Hospital College London, London, UK
e-mail: kolvekar@yahoo.com

N.L. Simon, MBBS
Department of School of Medical Education,
Kings College London, London, UK
e-mail: kolvekar@yahoo.com

S.K. Kolvekar, MBBS MS, MCh, FRCPS,
FRCS(CTh) (✉)
Department of Cardiothoracic Surgery,
University College London Hospitals, The Heart
Hospital and Barts Heart Center, London, UK
e-mail: kolvekar@yahoo.com

© Springer International Publishing Switzerland 2016
S.K. Kolvekar, H.K. Pilegaard (eds.), *Chest Wall Deformities and Corrective Procedures*,
DOI 10.1007/978-3-319-23968-2_14

Introduction

Acquired deformities of the chest wall are defined as malformations resulting from non-congenital causative factors. Acquired chest wall deformities account for less than 1 % of all thoracic wall malformations [1]. In contrast to the low incidence of acquired chest wall malformations, a wide variety of causative factors as well as clinical manifestations and presentations have been identified. Treatment strategies therefore vary significantly and must be tailored in accordance to the causative pathology and extend of the condition.

The large spectrum of underlying causes and manifestations of these deformities have made a comprehensive description and classification difficult and consequently only a limited volume of literature has been published. Fokin and Robicsek proposed in 2006 a classification of acquired chest wall deformities based on etiology [1]. The original publication focused on malformations of the anterior chest wall, however the classification can be applied in minor modification to the entire spectrum of acquired thoracic wall deformities.

Classification of acquired chest wall deformities, modified after Fokin and Robicsek:

1. Deformities, which developed as result of a primary disease of the chest wall
2. Iatrogenic deformities caused by surgical intervention to the chest wall
3. Traumatic deformities resulting from direct or indirect injury to the chest

Chest Wall Deformities Due to Primary Disease of the Chest Wall

The thoracic wall comprises of multiple layers of anatomical structures, including skin, subcutaneous fat tissue, fasciae, muscles, bones, cartilages, joints, parietal pleura and neurovascular structures. A disease process of any thoracic wall structures, typically infection or tumor may result in the development of a chest wall deformity.

Bacterial or fungal infections of the chest wall are more frequently found in the adult than in the pediatric patient population. Fungal infections are more common in the immunosuppressed patient. Infections of the chest wall develop following hematogenous spread or due to direct extension and present as myositis, fasciitis or osteomyelitis. Abscess formation and tissue destruction can lead to subsequent deformation of the thoracic wall. Staphylococcus aureus has been identified as responsible microorganism with the highest prevalence [2]. Destructive chest wall infections have also been encountered due to Mycobateria, Salmonella, Actinomyces, Aspergillus and Candida species [2–4]. Local signs of infection such as erythema, swelling, fistula or pain but also the appearance of an asymptomatic chest wall mass should always prompt an investigation for an infectious cause. Ultrasound, CT and MR scanning are diagnostic tools of choice [5]. Identification of the responsible pathogen is paramount to guide the antimicrobial treatment.

Benign and malignant tumor growth may develop within the thoracic wall affecting cartilaginous, osseous and/or soft tissue. Due to their aggressive nature, malignant tumors often involve multiple layers of the chest wall. Chest wall tumors are an overall infrequent disease but present a wide range of pathologies. Diagnosis and treatment are guided by oncological principles.

During infancy and childhood, tumors of the chest wall are rare findings but if encountered, usually malignant [6]. The Ewing sarcoma family of tumors are the most frequently found malignant tumors of the chest wall in children [7]. Rhabdomyosarcoma is the second most common pediatric chest wall malignancy with a typical poor prognosis [8]. Rare chest wall malignancies among children are thoracic lymphoma, neuroblastoma, congenital fibrosarcoma, mesenchymal chondrosarcoma, osteosarcoma [9] and malignant peripheral nerve sheath tumors (Figs. 14.1 and 14.2) [5].

Most common benign chest wall tumors in infants and children are lymphangiomas, hemangiomas and mixed lymphangiohemangiomas. These often cystic tumors are typically located within the chest wall, axilla or neck and can increase rapidly in size due to spontaneous intracapsular hemorrhage. Benign soft tissue tumors affecting the thoracic wall during infancy and childhood are lipoblastoma, neurofibromatosis and

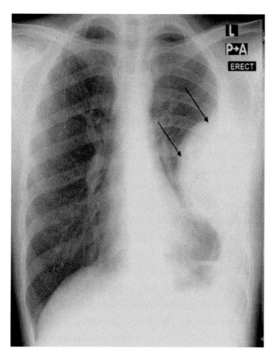

Fig. 14.1 Chest radiograph showing a large pleural-based mass in the left hemithorax (*arrows*), with underlying rib destruction and a pleural effusion (From Lim et al. [9] This is an open-access article distributed under the terms of the Creative Commons Attribution License, which permits unrestricted use, distribution, and reproduction in any medium, provided the original work is properly cited)

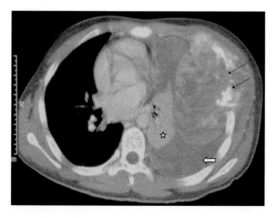

Fig. 14.2 A contrast enhanced CT examination of the chest showing a large heterogenously enhancing solid mass arising from the skeletal chest wall with lytic destruction of the rib and calcifications (*arrows*). There is a moderate-sized pleural effusion (*block arrow*) and underlying lung collapse and consolidation (*star*) (From Lim et al. [9] This is an open-access article distributed under the terms of the Creative Commons Attribution License, which permits unrestricted use, distribution, and reproduction in any medium, provided the original work is properly cited)

fibrous tumors (fibroma, fibromatosis, fibrous hamartoma). Ribs, vertebrae, clavicle, scapula and sternum can be affected by osteochondromas as solitary or multiple lesions. Neurogenic chest wall tumors (schwannomas, neurofibromas) arise from intercostal nerves or sympatic ganglia and may lead to destruction of adjacent rips or vertebrae [5].

The majority of chest wall neoplasms in the adult patient population are malignant metastatic disease from either distant carcinomas or sarcomas, or due to direct invasion from adjacent thoracic malignancies of lung, pleura, mediastinum or breast [10].

Primary malignant chest wall tumors are rare findings, representing only 1–2 % of all primary tumors [11] and account for less than 1/3 of all chest wall neoplasms in the adult. The chest wall chondrosarcoma is the most common primary thoracic wall tumor, typically located in the anterior chest wall, arising parasternal from the costochondral junction or the sternum itself [12]. Osteosarcomas of the chest wall are rare. Although the osteosarcoma is the most common primary malignant tumor of the bone, only 3 % originate from the chest wall [13]. Ewing's sarcomas are typically found in children, however 1/3 of cases encountered, affect patients above the age of 20 years. Further primary chest wall tumors reported in adult patients are plasmacytoma, soft tissue sarcoma and lymphoma. Radiation associated malignancies of the chest wall (malignant fibrous histiocytoma, radiation-induced sarcomas) may develop regardless of the original primary tumor and should be treated as de novo tumor [14].

Due to the rarity of primary chest wall tumors, most series published are of limited case numbers. Primary benign chest wall tumors have been reported to account for 21–67 % in various studies [10]. Osteochondroma and chondromas are the most common benign tumors. Lipoma is the most common benign soft tissue tumor. Benign tumors may cause significant chest wall deformities due to mass effect [15].

Iatrogenic Chest Wall Deformities

Iatrogenic deformities of the chest wall represent malformations which develop secondarily following a surgical intervention to the chest wall such as open repair of congenital pectus deformities, harvesting of rip grafts or inadequate closure of thoracotomies.

Surgical correction of pectus excavatum deformities involved originally various degrees of rip and cartilage resection. First surgical repair, with partial unilateral resection of 2nd and 3rd rip segments, was reported in 1911 by Ludwig Meyer [16]. His patient, however, suffered early recurrence of the deformity and associated respiratory symptoms [17]. Sauerbruch undertook in 1913 the first successful surgical repair of a pectus excavatum with satisfactory long-term result, performing a more extensive unilateral chondrocostal resection of the 5th to 9th rip with partial sternectomy [18]. The principle foundation of pectus surgery, on which all later on developed surgical techniques have orientated on, is attributed to Lexer and Hofmeister, who described in 1927 a technique of pectus excavatum repair involving bilateral chondrocostal resection with mobilization of the sternum [17]. This technique was developed further by Ravitch and published in 1949 [19]. The Ravitch procedure requires the excision of all deformed costal cartilages including pericondrium. Modifications of the Ravitch technique were reported by Welch and Shamberger [20, 21] and Robicsek [22–24] and remain basis for current open repair of the pectus excavatum deformity (Fig. 14.3a–c).

During the early and mid 1990s, the attention of the surgical society was directed at a group of young patients who presented with symptoms of severe respiratory distress during minimal exercise and universal physical finding of a small and narrow thorax with immobile chest wall and primary diaphragmatic breathing [25, 26]. All these patients, typically children and teenagers were in common a past medical history of extensive open repair of a pectus excavatum deformity during early childhood before the age of 4 years. None of the patients showed recurrence of the pectus deformity, however all had developed a reduced and restricted thorax with debilitating restrictive pulmonary disorder. Pulmonary function showed significantly decreased vital capacity and forced expiratory volume with impaired exercise capacity and desaturations during exercise [25, 26].

A history of recurrent episodes of pneumonia requiring hospitalization was common. Radiographic imaging identified markedly reduced sagittal and transverse diameters of the chest with low-lying diaphragm [1, 26]. The sternum was often atrophic, short and depressed. Para-sternal fusion of rips was common finding [27]. This restrictive chest wall condition following pectus repair was termed "acquired Jeune's syndrome" due to the striking similarity of findings with the asphyxiating thoracic chondrodystrophy or Jeune's syndrome [25]. Jeuen's syndrome is a rare autosomal recessive disorder affecting the development of bone and cartilage with subsequent skeletal dysplasia [28]. Thoracic cage growth retardation with pulmonary hypoplasia leads frequently to death during infancy due to respiratory insufficiency. With improved postnatal management, patients may survive to childhood or early adolescence [29]. As the complex of Jeune's syndrome extends beyond the chest wall anatomy, Robicsek introduced the term of "acquired restrictive thoracic dystrophy" (ARTD) to describe the complication of a restricted and dystrophic chest cage following extensive pectus excavatum deformity repair [30]. A uniform terminology has not yet been agreed on. Authors continue to use multiple terms, such as "acquired restrictive thoracic dystrophy (ARTD)" [30], "acquired asphyxiating thoracic dystrophy [31, 32], "acquired thoracic dystrophy" [33] or "acquired Jeune's syndrome" [27].

Thoracic growth retardation in ARTD is a direct result of surgical trauma to the costochondral growth plates or of their resection at young age, with the degree of ARDT severity depending upon the extent of cartilage extirpation [1]. Injury or resection of the costochondral growth centers prevents normal development and growth of the rip cage. Experimental studies have identified the sternal costochondral junction as the site where most of the longitudinal growth of the rib takes place as a result of endochondrial bone formation [34, 35]. During infancy, when compared to childhood, a significantly higher number of cells and proportion of proliferative chondrocytes are present at the sternal costochondral junction [36]. Excision of costal cartilages without preservation of the costal growth centers severely affects the

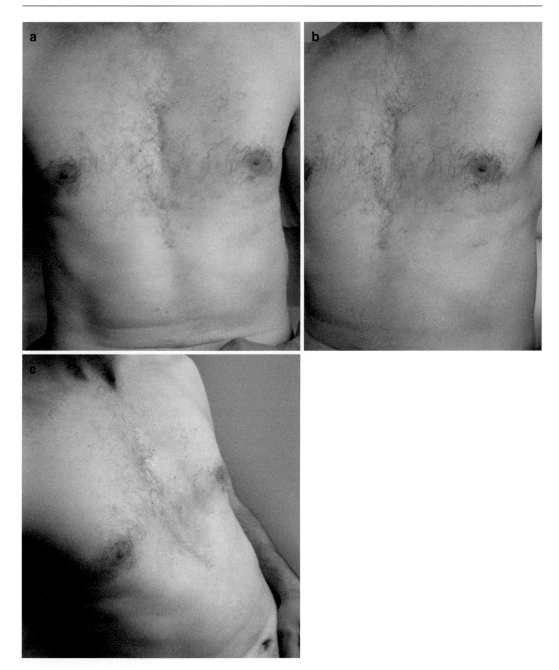

Fig. 14.3 (**a**) Sternal depression after Ravitch procedure; (**b**) Sternal depression after Ravitch procedure left side view; (**c**) Sternal depression after Ravitch procedure right side view

transvers and sagittal thoracic development as shown in experimental studies by Martinez et al. [37] and Calik et al. [38]. In addition, further restriction of the chest can be caused by retrosternal suturing of rips or perichondral sheaths as additional sternal support, a technique introduced during the 1970s as adjunctive maneuver to prevent recurrence of sternal depression [39]. However, fibrosis and cartilage regeneration with subsequent ossification leads to formation of restrictive and fixed sub sternal plane, resulting in a frozen thorax [40]. Not only thoracic growth retardation with reduction in size, but also a severely impaired mobility and fixation of the chest wall is responsible for the observed cardiopulmonary effects in ARTD patients [25, 33].

The treatment of the acquired Jeune's syndrome remains a surgical challenge and is aimed to improve functional lung capacity by increasing the overall thoracic volume. A low-lying diaphragm and predominant diaphragmatic breathing are common findings. Improvement of pulmonary function may be achieved by enlargement of the thoracic cage with subsequent improved diaphragmatic respiration. Extensive and aggressive reconstruction of the chest wall is required in most cases. Reconstructive techniques in children often require multiple and staged procedures to enable progressive expansion of the chest during the child's growth. A number of techniques have been described. Due to the rarity of the condition, the published series consist of limited number of cases and further modifications of surgical techniques and strategies are to be expected.

In his landmark report on restrictive thoracic dystrophy following corrective pectus surgery at early age, which was the first report of its kind, Haller described during his presentation in 1995 a technique of anterior chest wall enlargement consisting of sternal mobilization with resection of the degenerated fibro-osseous sternocostal junction. The sternum was then elevated and fixed using multiple modified Rehbein splints [25].

Surgical experience gained in the treatment of the congenital Jeune's syndrome was transferred into the operative management of the acquired Jeune's syndrome. Barnes and Hull, surgeons at London's Great Ormond Street Hospital described in 1971 a technique of thoracic volume enlargement for children with congenital Jeune's syndrome, involving a median sternotomy and splinting of the sternum using autologous bone graft and bone matrix [41]. This surgical technique has since been refined and recommended for its simplicity, short operating time, and effectiveness [42, 43]. At the St Louis' Cardinal Glennon Children's Hospital, Weber adopted Barnes' technique for his ARTD patients. Weber and colleagues reported in 1998 their first case of ARTD correction using the technique of sternal midline split with permanent separation of the sternal halves by rip graft interposition [31]. Additional rib cage enlargement was achieved by bilateral rip resection. In 2005, Weber's group published a further report on a total of ten patients treated by the method described above with overall satisfactory functional results [32].

In 2014, Paul Colombani's group of the John Hopkins Hospital published their experience and surgical approach [27]. Between 1996 and 2011, 19 patients (aged 11–37 years) underwent extensive chest wall reconstruction for ARTD following Ravitch procedure at a mean age of 4.63 years. Sufficient re-expansion of the chest cage was achieved by repeated modified Ravitch procedure in two patients. The remaining 17 patients required extensive reconstructive surgery to achieve expansion of the thoracic cage by mobilization and elevation of the sternum and complete reconstruction of the anterior chest wall. Thorough exposure of the anterior thoracic cage was achieved by mobilization of bilateral pectoralis muscle flaps and separation of the rectus abdominis muscle from the xyphoid through a transvers anterior chest wall incision. Mobilization of the sternum was achieved by bilateral transection of the parasternal fibrous scar tissue and resection of deformed cartilages. A transvers anterior osteotomy at the sterno-manubrial junction was made to allow elevation of the corpus sterni by wiring the corpus onto the top edge of the manubrium. The costosternal continuity was restored by wiring of the lower cartilages to the sternum to improve stability of the anterior chest wall. Reconstruction of the costosternal margin in the absence of cartilages required utilization of autologous rip graft or femur allograft. Bilateral thoracic expansion gaps were created by serial rip osteotomies to allow further release of the anterior chest wall. One or two Lorenz bars were placed for retrosternal support.

A similar surgical technique, applied to adult ARTD patients, was reported in 2014 by Jaroszewski and co-workers from the Mayo Clinic Hospital in Phoenix [33]. Their patient collective consisted of nine male patients with a mean age of 34 years (range 22–42 years), who all underwent a Ravitch procedure for correction of pectus excavatum deformity between their 4th and 6th year of life. The operative approach involved the full mobilization of the sternum with multiple parasternal and lateral rip osteotomies to allow for anterior expansion of the thoracic cage and elevation of the sternum. Sternal support was provided with a Lorenz bar. Multiple Titanium plates were used to stabilize the sternal osteotomy and lateral chest wall. The sternocostal junctions were reconstructed using Polyglactin mesh and bone matrix.

Operative and functional outcome of ARTD surgery are encouraging. Although the chest wall reconstructions are complex procedures with significant potential intra- and postoperative complications, a successful repair can be performed safely. The majority of patients reported a subjective improvement in preoperative symptoms, ability to exercise and quality of life [27, 32, 33]. Postoperative improvement of measurable pulmonary function is however modest only [27], emphasizing the severity of permanent thoracic organ dysfunction due to persistent limitation of thoracic wall excursion and ceased growth development caused by the condition.

Prevention of ARTD as complication of corrective pectus surgery is adamant. All reported patients suffering from ARTD underwent a Ravitch-type operation at a very young age. It was therefore quickly advocated that open surgical correction of a pectus deformity should be delayed until skeletal growth and development are completed. However, Robicsek argued that pectus surgery can be performed safely even at young age as long the essential principle of limited cartilagous resection ensuring preservation of the costochondral growth centres in not violated [22, 30]. A segment of cartilage should be preserved at the sternal and costal end. The posterior perichondrium should be preserved in its entire length to allow for chondral regeneration. Retrosternal suturing of perichondrium or rips must be avoided as this manoeuvre has been shown to contribute significantly to thoracic constriction due to fibrosis and ossification. Robicsek concluded that "the solution to the problem of preventing the development of acquired restric-

tive thoracic dystrophy after pectus excavatum repair is not to delay surgical intervention, but to do it appropriately." [1]

Other forms of iatrogenic chest wall malformations are pectus deformities, which develop after surgical intervention involving the sternum or anterior chest wall. Most common are acquired pectus carinatum deformities, evolving several years postoperatively [44, 45]. The initial surgery often over-corrected an existing pectus excavatum deformity. Development of an iatrogenic pectus carinatum has also been observed following median sternotomy for cardiac surgery in early childhood [46]. A carinatum-type deformity has been reported after corrective surgery for sternal cleft malformation [45]. The "floating sternum" describes an unstable anterior chest wall with chronic and persistent complete detachment of the sternum from all costochondral junctions [40]. This complication of pectus excavatum repair has been observed years after the initial surgery and is understood to be caused by extensive resection of the costal cartilages and perichondrium or failure of proper regeneration of resected cartilages [47].

Iatrogenic chest wall deformities have been well documented after harvesting of costal cartilage for ear reconstruction [48, 49]. Two types of deformity have been recognized, chest wall depression deformity and costal arch deformity. The incidence of both deformities is significantly higher among male patients, after cartilage harvest from the upper rips and in patients younger than 10 years of age at the time of surgery. Development of a thoracic scoliosis following rip graft harvesting has also been observed [48].

Lung herniation is a further form of chest wall deformity. Although lung hernias are usually congenital, spontaneous or traumatic in origin [50], a growing body of evidence has been published over the recent years, reporting cases of postoperative lung herniations directly related to the surgical access to the chest. Lung hernias have been observed after minimal invasive cardiac surgery or lung transplantation [51–54]. In the effort of limiting the surgical incision, the actual length of intercostal space division often exceeds significantly the skin incision, which may be a contributing factor for insufficient closure of the intercostal space. Iatrogenic postoperative lung hernias are a result of insufficient closure or failed healing of a thoracotomy. Patients present with a localized chest wall swelling and often pleuritic pain at the side of previous surgery. The herniation of the lung may present as persistent or intermittent chest wall bulge, related to respiration and typically provokable by Valsalva maneuver. Herniorrhaphy can be safely accomplished via thoracoscopic access, employing direct or patch closure of the chest wall defect [50, 55]. Indication for repair is given in all cases of iatrogenic lung hernias as they may lead to complications such as life-threatening hemorrhage [54, 56].

Traumatic Chest Wall Deformities

Direct trauma to the torso may lead to a wide spectrum of chest wall injuries and deformities. Falls and road traffic accidents are among the most common causes of chest and chest wall injuries. Fractures of single of multiple rips are the most frequent type of chest wall injury [57]. Fracture of single or non-consecutive rips will usually not require surgical intervention, however misalignment and malfusion can result in significant chest wall deformation. Extensive rip fractures may result in a mechanically unstable, flail chest, associated with significant rates of short-term mortality and long-term morbidity, especially among the elderly population [58]. The definition of the flail chest is not uniform throughout the literature. Most common definition is of an unilateral fracture of three or more consecutive ribs in at least two locations, creating a flail chest wall segment [57]. Various techniques of flail chest wall stabilization and reconstruction have been described, such as Kirschner wires, Judet's struts, polypropylene mesh, titanium plates or Lorenz bars [59].

Sternal fractures are a result of direct traumatic impact to the anterior chest wall or flexion-compression injury of the trunk. Extensive trauma to the anterior chest wall may lead due to sternal and costal fractures to the development of a flail anterior chest wall segment. Without adequate surgical reconstruction and stabilization, pseudo articulations or post-traumatic pectus excavatum and carinatum deformities may develop [1, 60].

References

1. Fokin AA, Robicsek F. Acquired deformities of the anterior chest wall. Thorac Cardiovasc Surg. 2006; 54(1):57–61.
2. Wong K-S, Hung IJ, Wang CR, Lien R. Thoracic wall lesions in children. Pediatr Pulmonol. 2004;37(3): 257–63.
3. Sakran W, Bisharat N. Primary chest wall abscess caused by Escherichia coli costochondritis. Am J Med Sci. 2011;342(3):241–6.
4. Aharmim M, Kouismi H, Marc K, Soualhi M, Zahraoui R, Benamor J, et al. Pulmonary actinomycosis with chest wall fistula formation in a child. Arch Pediatr. 2014;21(7):757–60.
5. García-Peña P, Barber I. Pathology of the thoracic wall: congenital and acquired. Pediatr Radiol. 2010; 40(6):859–68.
6. Shamberger RC, Grier HE. Chest wall tumors in infants and children. Semin Pediatr Surg. 1994;3(4): 267–76.
7. Shamberger RC, Tarbell NJ, Perez-Atayde AR, Grier HE. Malignant small round cell tumor (Ewing's-PNET) of the chest wall in children. J Pediatr Surg. 1994;29(2):179–84; discussion 184–5.
8. Saenz NC, Ghavimi F, Gerald W, Gollamudi S, LaQuaglia MP. Chest wall rhabdomyosarcoma. Cancer [Internet]. 1997;80(8):1513–7 [cited 22 Jan 2015].
9. Lim WY, Ahmad Sarji S, Yik YI, Ramanujam TM. Osteosarcoma of the rib. Biomed Imaging Intervention J. 2008;4(1), e7.
10. Chudacek J, Bohanes T, Szkorupa M, Klein J, Stasek M, Zalesak B, et al. Strategies of treatment of chest wall tumors and our experience. Rozhl Chir. 2015; 94(1):17–23.
11. Weyant MJ, Bains MS, Venkatraman E, Downey RJ, Park BJ, Flores RM, et al. Results of chest wall resection and reconstruction with and without rigid prosthesis. Ann Thorac Surg. 2006;81(1):279–85.
12. Fong Y-C, Pairolero PC, Sim FH, Cha SS, Blanchard CL, Scully SP. Chondrosarcoma of the chest wall: a retrospective clinical analysis. Clin Orthop Relat Res. 2004;427:184–9.
13. Gladish GW, Sabloff BM, Munden RF, Truong MT, Erasmus JJ, Chasen MH. Primary thoracic sarcomas. Radiographics. 2002;22(3):621–37.
14. Schwarz RE, Burt M. Radiation-associated malignant tumors of the chest wall. Ann Surg Oncol. 1996;3(4): 387–92.
15. Pop D, Venissac N, Mouroux J. Remodelling acquired chest wall deformity after removal of a large axillary lipoma. Interact Cardiovasc Thorac Surg. 2010;10(1):105–6.

16. Meyer L. Zur chirurgischen Behandlung der angeborenen Trichterbrust. Berl Klin Wschr. 1911;48:1563–6.
17. BRUCK H, LORBEK W. Surgical treatment of congenital funnel chest. Langenbecks Arch Klin Chir Ver Dtsch Z Chir. 1956;281(5):465–71.
18. Sauerbruch F. Chirurgie der Brustorgane. 2nd ed. Berlin: Springer; 1920.
19. Ravitch MM. The operative treatment of pectus excavatum. Ann Surg. 1949;129(4):429–44.
20. WELCH KJ. Satisfactory surgical correction of pectus excavatum deformity in childhood; a limited opportunity. J Thorac Surg. 1958;36(5):697–713.
21. Shamberger RC, Welch KJ. Surgical repair of pectus excavatum. J Pediatr Surg. 1988;23(7):615–22.
22. Robicsek F, Watts LT, Fokin AA. Surgical repair of pectus excavatum and carinatum. Semin Thorac Cardiovasc Surg. 2009;21(1):64–75.
23. Robicsek F, Fokin A. Surgical correction of pectus excavatum and carinatum. J Cardiovasc Surg (Torino). 1999;40(5):725–31.
24. Robicsek F. Marlex mesh support for the correction of very severe and recurrent pectus excavatum. Ann Thorac Surg. 1978;26(1):80–3.
25. Haller JA, Colombani PM, Humphries CT, Azizkhan RG, Loughlin GM. Chest wall constriction after too extensive and too early operations for pectus excavatum. Ann Thorac Surg. 1996;61(6):1618–24; discussion 1625.
26. Milović I, Oluić D. The effect of the age of the child at the time of surgery for pectus excavatum on respiratory function and anthropometric parameters of the thorax. Acta Chir Iugosl. 1990;37(1):45–52.
27. Sacco Casamassima MG, Goldstein SD, Salazar JH, Papandria D, McIltrot KH, O'Neill DE, et al. Operative management of acquired Jeune's syndrome. J Pediatr Surg. 2014;49(1):55–60; discussion 60.
28. O'Connor MB, Gallagher DP, Mulloy E. Jeune syndrome. Postgrad Med J. 2008;84(996):559.
29. De Vries J, Yntema JL, van Die CE, Crama N, Cornelissen EAM, Hamel BCJ. Jeune syndrome: description of 13 cases and a proposal for follow-up protocol. Eur J Pediatr. 2010;169(1):77–88.
30. Robicsek F, Fokin AA. How not to do it: restrictive thoracic dystrophy after pectus excavatum repair. Interact Cardiovasc Thorac Surg. 2004;3(4):566–8.
31. Weber TR, Kurkchubasche AG. Operative management of asphyxiating thoracic dystrophy after pectus repair. J Pediatr Surg. 1998;33(2):262–5.
32. Weber TR. Further experience with the operative management of asphyxiating thoracic dystrophy after pectus repair. J Pediatr Surg. 2005;40(1):170–3.
33. Jaroszewski DE, Notrica DM, McMahon LE, Hakim FA, Lackey JJ, Gruden JF, et al. Operative management of acquired thoracic dystrophy in adults after open pectus excavatum repair. Ann Thorac Surg. 2014;97(5):1764–70.
34. Peltomäki T, Häkkinen L. Growth of the ribs at the costochondral junction in the rat. J Anat. 1992;181(Pt 2):259–64.
35. Snellman O. Growth and remodelling of the ribs in normal and scoliotic pigs. Acta Orthop Scand Suppl. 1973;149:1–85.
36. Gruber HE, Rimoin DL. Quantitative histology of cartilage cell columns in the human costochondral junction: findings in newborn and pediatric subjects. Pediatr Res. 1989;25(2):202–4.
37. Martinez D, Juame J, Stein T, Peña A. The effect of costal cartilage resection on chest wall development. Pediatr Surg Int. 1990;5(3):170–3.
38. Calik M, Aribas OK, Kanat F. The effect of costal cartilage resection on the chest wall development: a morphometric evaluation. Eur J Cardiothorac Surg. 2007;32(5):756–60.
39. Fonkalsrud EW, Follette D, Sarwat AK. Pectus excavatum repair using autologous perichondrium for sternal support. Arch Surg. 1978;113(12):1433–7.
40. Colombani PM. Recurrent chest wall anomalies. Semin Pediatr Surg. 2003;12(2):94–9.
41. Barnes ND, Hull D, Milner AD, Waterston DJ. Chest reconstruction in thoracic dystrophy. Arch Dis Child. 1971;46(250):833–7.
42. Todd DW, Tinguely SJ, Norberg WJ. A thoracic expansion technique for Jeune's asphyxiating thoracic dystrophy. J Pediatr Surg. 1986;21(2):161–3.
43. Sharoni E, Erez E, Chorev G, Dagan O, Vidne BA. Chest reconstruction in asphyxiating thoracic dystrophy. J Pediatr Surg. 1998;33(10):1578–81.
44. Swanson JW, Colombani PM. Reactive pectus carinatum in patients treated for pectus excavatum. J Pediatr Surg. 2008;43(8):1468–73.
45. Bairov GA, Fokin AA. Keeled chest. Vestn Khir Im I I Grek. 1983;130(2):89–94.
46. Haje SA. Iatrogenic pectus carinatum. A case report. Int Orthop. 1995;19(6):370–3.
47. Prabhakaran K, Paidas CN, Haller JA, Pegoli W, Colombani PM. Management of a floating sternum after repair of pectus excavatum. J Pediatr Surg. 2001;36(1):159–64.
48. Ohara K, Nakamura K, Ohta E. Chest wall deformities and thoracic scoliosis after costal cartilage graft harvesting. Plast Reconstr Surg. 1997;99(4):v1030–6.
49. Guo W-H, Yang Q-H, Jiang H-Y, Zhuang H-X. Clinical study of chest contour deformity after harvesting of costal cartilage for total ear reconstruction. Zhonghua Zheng Xing Wai Ke Za Zhi. 2008;24(5):365–7.
50. Seder CW, Allen MS, Nichols FC, Wigle DA, Shen KR, Deschamps C, et al. Primary and prosthetic repair of acquired chest wall hernias: a 20-year experience. Ann Thorac Surg. 2014;98(2):484–9.
51. Fiscon V, Portale G, Frigo F, Migliorini G. Thoracoscopic repair of lung herniation following minimally invasive cardiothoracic surgery. Chir Ital. 2009;61(2):261–3.
52. Athanassiadi K, Bagaev E, Simon A, Haverich A. Lung herniation: a rare complication in minimally invasive cardiothoracic surgery. Eur J Cardiothorac Surg. 2008;33(5):774–6.

53. Santini M, Fiorello A, Vicidomini G, Busiello L. Pulmonary hernia secondary to limited access for mitral valve surgery and repaired by video thoracoscopic surgery. Interact Cardiovasc Thorac Surg. 2009;8(1):111–3.

54. Schroeter T, Bittner H, Subramanian S, Hänsig M, Mohr F, Borger M. Life-threatening hemothorax resulting from lung hernia after minimally invasive mitral valve surgery. Thorac Cardiovasc Surg. 2011; 59(4):252–4.

55. Mirza A, Gogna R, Kumaran M, Malik M, Martin-Ucar A. The surgical management of intercostal lung herniation using bioprosthesis. J Surg Case Rep. 2011;2011(2):6.

56. Emberger JS, Racine L, Maheshwari V. Lung hernia associated with hemothorax following cardiopulmo-nary resuscitation. Respir Care [Internet]. 2011;56(7):1037–9 [cited 29 Jan 2015].

57. Lafferty PM, Anavian J, Will RE, Cole PA. Operative treatment of chest wall injuries: indications, technique, and outcomes. J Bone Joint Surg Am [Internet]. 2011;93(1):97–110 [cited 22 Dec 2014].

58. Vodicka J, Spidlen V, Safránek J, Simánek V, Altmann P. Severe injury to the chest wall--experience with surgical therapy. Zentralbl Chir [Internet]. 2007;132(6):542–6 [cited 29 Jan 2015].

59. Lee SA, Hwang JJ, Chee HK, Kim YH, Lee WS. Flail chest stabilization with Nuss operation in presence of multiple myeloma. J Thorac Dis [Internet]. 2014;6(5):E43–7 [cited 20 Jan 2015].

60. Alexander J. Traumatic pectus excavatum. Ann Surg. 1931;93(2):489–500 [cited 29 Jan 2015].

Revision of Prior Failed/Recurrent Pectus Excavatum Surgery

15

Dawn E. Jaroszewski and Kevin J. Johnson

Abstract

Recurrence of pectus excavatum deformities occurs after both open and MIRPE. Recurrence risks are also based on multiple factors and differ based on the initial repair procedure. Identifying the contributing factors to a previous procedure's failure is critical to proper repair and prevention of another recurrence. Each case must be taken on an individual basis and is contingent on the patient's anatomy and previous repair technique. A combination of surgical techniques may be necessary in to successful repair some patients.

Keywords

Pectus Excavatum • Ravitch • Nuss • Complications • Recurrence • Failure • Revision surgery

Background

Surgical repair of pectus excavatum (PE) has evolved significantly over the past 50 years. There are a variety of techniques that have been successfully used on patients of all ages but the two most common methods used today include modifications of the open Ravitch approach and

D.E. Jaroszewski, MD, MBA, FACS (✉)
Department of Cardiothoracic Surgery,
Mayo Clinic Arizona, Phoenix, AZ, USA
e-mail: Jaroszewski.dawn@mayo.edu

K.J. Johnson, MD
Department of General Surgery,
Mayo Clinic Arizona, Phoenix, AZ, USA

the minimally invasive repair (MIRPE) or "Nuss". Recurrence rates after repair of PE using both techniques have been reported in 2–37 % of patients [1–17]. No high-quality reports comparing long-term recurrences of MIRPE to open repair have been published. The cause of recurrence varies based on the technique of initial repair utilized. For patients presenting after failed or recurrent primary MIRPE repair; the placement, number of bars, bar migration, and too early of support removal can all be associated with failure (Figs. 15.1a, b and 15.2a, b) [2, 4, 12–14, 18–28]. Connective tissue disorders can complicate and increase recurrence risk in both previous Nuss and open PE repairs [1, 4, 29, 30]. Recurrence risks for the open repair are also

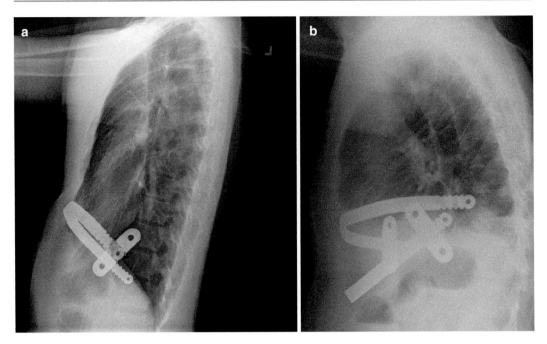

Fig. 15.1 (**a, b**) Failure of the Nuss procedure can be due to bar rotation or migration as is seen in these two patient's lateral chest roentgenogram (**a**) rotation of a long bar with single stabilizers is seen, (**b**) Rotation of the lower bar is seen on this patient with 2 support bars and stabilizers

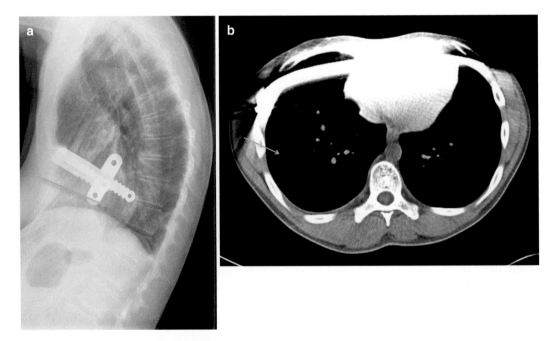

Fig. 15.2 Too lateral entrance of the support bars positions the support bars intrathoracic and fails to elevate the defect anteriorly. (**a**) posteriorly displaced bar is seen on in this patient's lateral chest roentgenogram. *Arrow* point to pectus excavatum defect still seen below the level of the bar. (**b**) computerized tomography shows intrathoracic portion of support bar with failure to support and elevate the pectus excavatum defect. *Arrow* points to the space between the chest wall and the bar

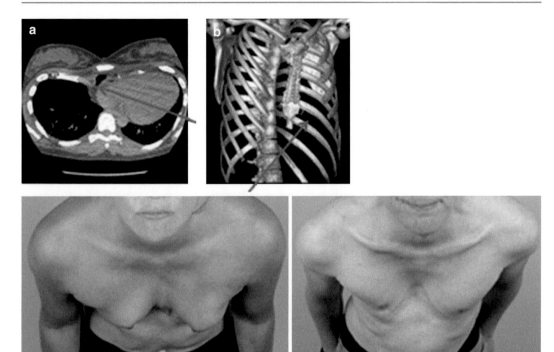

Fig. 15.3 Malunion and recurrence of pectus excavatum defect after previous Ravitch repair are seen in these patient's photographs, computerized tomography and 3-D reconstruction images (**a**) A 46 year-old female with significant recurrence after open Ravitch procedure. CT scan shows failed union between the rib (*thin arrow*) and Sternum (*thick arrow*) (**b**) A 44 year old male with significant recurrence after open Ravitch procedure. 3D reconstruction shows recurrence and failure of the chest wall to reconstitute

based on multiple factors which include incomplete previous repair, repair at a young age, dissection either too extensive or too little, early removal or lack of support structures, and incomplete healing of the chest wall with pseudoarthrosis and necrosis (Fig. 15.3a, b) [1, 3, 5, 8, 13–15, 16, 21, 31–34, 35, 36].

Regardless of which initial procedure was used, some patients will experience recurrence. There are only a few publications devoted exclusively to repair of recurrent pectus deformities, and most studies include children with only a few adults [1–5, 9, 11, 13, 14, 31, 37]. Several of these publications are reviewed in Table 15.1. Most of these reports describe experience with a single operative technique in the repair of recurrent pectus excavatum. The reports by Redlinger and Croitoru et al. advocated a modified Nuss technique for both open and Nuss recurrent PE [13, 14]. Multiple bars were required and they reported slightly higher complication and bar dis-

placement rates with revision versus primary repairs. Others have advocated the use of a modified open Ravitch repair in all patients with recurrent PE, reporting excellent results in a small group of patients, with only a marginally longer length of stay compared to patients undergoing primary repair (6 days versus 5 days) [9]. Studies have shown that repairs in adults may be more difficult and have increased risks of complications due to increased rigidity of the chest wall [3, 7, 10, 18, 30, 31, 38–48]. Complex open repairs were required in many adult patients after prior open repair when compared to other studies [9, 32, 33]. Luu et al., reported on 13 recurrent patients in ages 16–54 years [9]. Eight of these were previous MIRPE and 5 had been a modified Ravitch repair. All of the failed MIRPE procedure patients in this series underwent a modified Ravitch repair for correction, while the recurrent open repair patients required complex reconstructions. Results are reported as good or excel-

Table 15.1 Publications for the surgical treatment of recurrent pectus excavatum

Author	# of patients	Median age at time of reoperation	Primary repair procedure (Nuss, open)	Operative technique secondary repair	Median operative time	Results reported	Length of follow-up (average)
Croitoru et al. [14]	50	16 years	Nuss 23 Open 27 Multiple 2	Minimally invasive Modified Nuss	140 min	8 % required revision surgery for bar displacement, 85 % report increased exercise tolerance post-op	NR
Liu et al. [31]	18	21 years	Nuss 1 Open 16 Other 1	Minimally invasive Modified Nuss	68.5 min	No bar displacement requiring reoperation, 14/18 (85 %) excellent result, 4/14 (15 %) good result	19 months
Miller et al. [11].	10	15 years		Minimally invasive Modified Nuss	70 min	Good or excellent results in all patients, no complications	23 months
Redlinger et al. [13].	100	17 years	Nuss 51 Open 45 Multiple 4	Minimally invasive Modified Nuss	NR	Bar displacement in 9 patients, 7 of which required reoperation, 2 intraoperative cardiac arrest	NR
Wang et al. [49].	12	15 years		Minimally invasive Modified Nuss	100 min	Bar displacement in 2 patients, no reoperation, excellent result in 66.7 %, good in 25 %, fair 8.3 %	10–38 months
Guo et al. [5].	28	15 years	Open 28	Minimally invasive Modified Nuss	86 min	Excellent results 64 %, Good 25 %, fair 11 %	24–72 months
Pison et al [64].				Minimally invasive Modified Nuss			
Luu et al. [9]	13	28 years	Nuss 8 Open 5	Nuss recurrences modified Ravitch Open recurrences required complex reconstruction not described	NR	1 patient returned to OR 2 years later for resection of protuberant costal cartilage, 10/13 excellent result, 2/13 good result	NR
Schulz-Drost et al. [34]		29 years	Open 7	Open revision with plating	205	High patient satisfaction results only	NR

lent in many patients undergoing reoperation [5, 9, 11, 31, 49]. Follow up is limited and the long-term durability of repairs unknown. Many publications do not report their length of follow up. Those studies that do provide a longer length of follow up have shown good efficacy in preventing further recurrence of PE during the follow-up periods [2, 5, 11, 31, 49].

Surgery for Recurrent Pectus Excavatum

In general, reoperative repair should avoid or repair the issues that contributed to the first surgical approach recurring. Assessment of why a patient's repair was unsuccessful or recurred is necessary for treating recurrence adequately. Both open and minimally invasive techniques have been described for repair of recurrent PE. Both approaches can offer advantages in the repair of recurrent defects, however, some recurrent defects may require an application of both open and minimally invasive repair techniques to achieve optimal outcomes. Regardless of the approach advocated, reports describing experience with repair of recurrent PE all mention the increased technical difficulties, higher complication rates and longer hospital stays [9, 11, 13, 14].

Recurrent Pectus Excavatum after MIRPE or Nuss Procedure

Recurrences following the Nuss repair are reported at a similar rate as that seen after Ravitch however many aspects of the presentation differ. Technical issues constitute a large proportion of the cases reported as "failed" versus "recurrent" in patients repaired with MIRPE. Some of the more common technical failures and causes reported for recurrent PE after Nuss procedure are listed in Table 15.2.

The majority of experienced centers reporting on revision of prior failed or recurrent MIRPE patients found that malpositioned or displaced bars were a large portion of the issue [2, 5, 13, 14, 31] (Fig. 15.4a–c). Bar displacement is the most

Table 15.2 Frequent causes of failed or recurrent prior MIRPE or Nuss procedure

Rotation or displacement of bars
Bars too long
Bars placed too lateral
Intercostal Stripping
Disproportionate weight distribution of chest wall on number of bars
Failure of bars to remain secured to chest wall
Failure to lift with bar placement
Chest wall too stiff and non-compliant
Adequate number of bars not utilized for weight & compliance of chest wall
Adequate number of bars not utilized for length and depth of defect
Bars stripped lateral failing to support chest anteriorly
Premature removal of bars
Connective tissue disorders

common complication following Nuss repair, with displacement rates greater than 10 % in some studies [6–8, 12, 19, 23, 25–27, 42, 43, 50–54]. Adult patients have also been noted to have a greater incidence of bar rotation and complications [4, 5]. This can lead to recurrence of the pectus deformity as well as need for subsequent reoperation. There are a variety of different issues that can lead to bar rotation and migration. The majority of revisions reported on noted bars that were too long (Fig. 15.5) [13, 14]. These bars were replaced with bars that were 1–4 in. shorter on average. Bars that were placed too lateral or intercostal stripping and lateral displacement occurring after placement was another common technical issue noted (Fig. 15.6a, b). When lateral displacement occurs, the bar will fail to contact the sternum and support it anteriorly (Fig. 15.7). The entry and exit sites into the chest should not be too lateral or muscle stripping can occur [13, 14, 20, 26, 53]. Use of a different interspace was recommended should intercostal stripping and lateral displacement occur [13]. Figure of eight suture reinforcement of the ribs bordering the stripped intercostal space can also be performed. The utilization of forced sternal elevation may also help facilitate bar placement and rotation and minimize intercostal stripping [55].

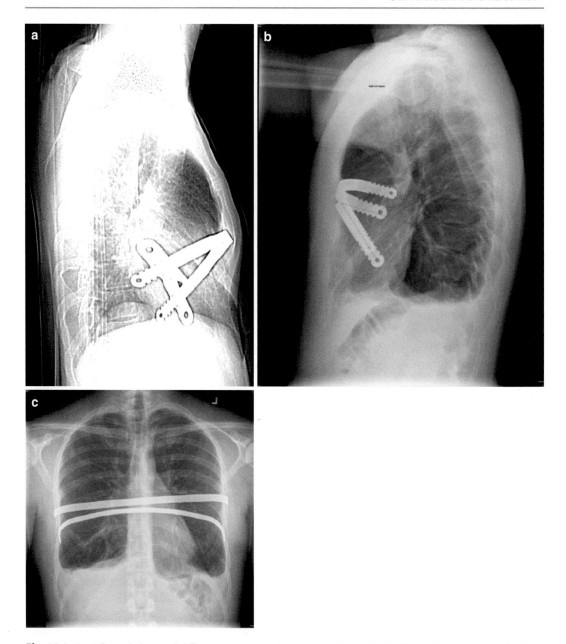

Fig. 15.4 (a–c) Lateral chest and A/P roentgenograms show bar rotation and migration in three patients after Nuss pectus excavatum repair

Adequate stability is also impacted by the number of bars and balance of the chest wall on support structures. For heavier, stiffer chests, several bars may be necessary to support the weight and elevate the defect. The pressure required to elevate the chest is significant and an inadequate number of bars to support the chest anterior can lead to lateral stripping of the intercostals and increased risk of bar rotation [22, 27, 55–58]. Recommendations as to what the adequate number of bars are varies [6, 18, 20, 25, 53, 59]. Initial reports of the Nuss procedure encompassed young patients with only one bar advocated however the majority recommend increased number of bars with more significant defects and advanced ages [53]. Older patients have also

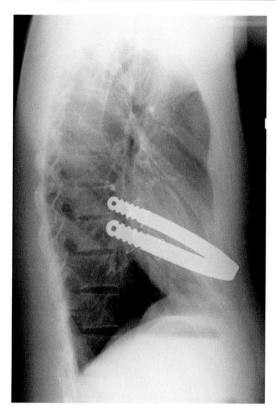

Fig. 15.5 Lateral roentgenogram of patient with recurrent pectus defect less than 1 month after Nuss repair and placement of single bar. Note a longer than recommended length of bar and curvature beyond the mid-axillary line with rotation and displacement

been reported by others to require more bars for PE repair and two or more bars may give better and more stable results [18, 25, 58, 60, 61]. For some patients presenting with reported recurrence, there may have been an incomplete repair of their defect following the initial Nuss with a portion of their defect remaining postsurgical due to an inadequate number of support bars (Fig. 15.8a–c) [3].

Recurrence has also been attributed to premature removal of the pectus bars before adequate remodeling has occurred and the chest wall secured into a corrected position. The optimal length of time recommended to leave support bars in place varies however, several experienced centers have increased their recommended time to 2–3 years [6, 7, 25, 40, 57, 62]. Patients with Marfan's and other connective tissue disorders

have been shown to have a higher risk for recurrence and recommendations are for leaving the bars in place for up to 4 years [1, 4, 29].

A significant problem encountered after a failed Nuss can be extensive intrathoracic adhesions [5]. These can require several hours of extensive adhesiolysis before dissection across the chest and mediastinum is achieved for bar placement. Use of sternal elevation may be helpful and others have described a subxiphoid incision to manually elevate the sternum during dissection across the chest, especially with extensive adhesions [5, 9, 13, 14, 63, 64].

Recurrent Pectus Excavatum after Ravitch and Open Procedures

The original open procedure for PE repair was described and accredited to Ravitch in the 1940s [65, 66]. Modifications of this technique have been used successfully for several decades [2, 15, 42, 67–69]. The open repair involves resection of the deformed costal cartilage with or without sternal osteotomy. Recurrence risks are based on multiple factors as listed in Table 15.3. Once recurrence occurs, subsequent repair becomes more complex. The challenges encountered with re-operative repair can vary based on the extent of initial operative repair. There is limited literature published on repair of recurrent open PE, however, most reported higher complication rates, longer hospital stays, and higher rates of bar displacement when repaired with MIRPE [5, 13, 14].

Surgical repair of patients having undergone a previous Ravitch or other open PE repair technique may have unique problems when recurrence occurs. Repair can be quite challenging due to rigidity of the bony chest wall and scar tissue from the prior surgical intervention. Extensive calcification, ossification and fusion of the previously excised cartilage may prevent adequate elevation of the chest wall without reexcision [9, 32, 33, 35, 70]. Osteotomies of the sternum, sterno-costal junctions and more laterally along the ribs may be necessary to mobilize the anterior chest wall. Recurrences following open PE repair

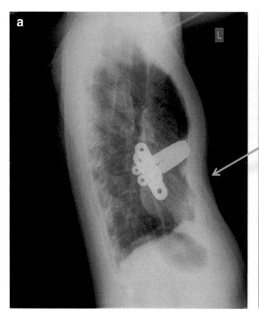
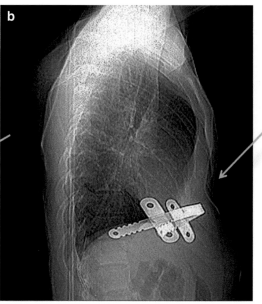

Fig. 15.6 (**a**, **b**) Lateral chest roentgenograms showing single pectus bar with failed elevation of the pectus excavatum defect secondary to lateral displacement (**a**) and intrathoracic migration (**b**). *Arrows* note pectus excavatum deformity still present despite support bar indwelling

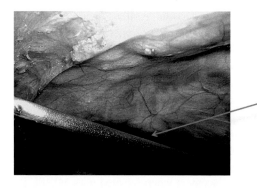

Fig. 15.7 Thoracoscopic view of intrathoracic pectus support bar which fails to contact the anterior chest wall due to lateral intercostal placement. *Arrow* notes space between chest wall and support bar

can also arise from osteonecrosis, malunion due to pseudomembranous attachments, instability and/or chest wall hernia (Fig. 15.9a, b) [1, 3, 4, 9, 17, 31, 33]. When non-union occurs bilaterally, this can also lead to an entity known as "floating sternum", which requires revision to reattach and stabilize the sternum (Fig. 15.10) [34, 36, 71].

Successful repair of areas of malunion, pseudo-arthrosis and sternal floating requires repeat open repair. Open repair and stabilization has also been recommended by other authors for these complicated recurrences [3, 9]. Rib/sternal reattachment and sites of repeated osteotomies prone to malunion or non-union can be approximated with titanium plating or Fiberwire™ (Arthrex, Inc, Naples, FL).

Rigidity of the chest wall following Ravitch is the main component that must be overcome to achieve an adequate repair. MIRPE is more difficult as a result, and bar displacement more likely. Additionally, a study by Redlinger et. al. also mentions findings of significant intrathoracic adhesions following Ravitch repair, despite this being considered an extra-pleural repair, making placement of pectus bars difficult [13]. The use of forced sternal elevation to move the sternum anterior has been reported to be helpful for safe dissection and repair with MIRPE [55, 57, 72–74].

Despite these challenges, MIRPE following previous open repair can be quite successful [5, 11, 14, 31]. Redlinger et al. reported on 100 patients they successfully repaired with the Nuss procedure after recurrences (45 prior open and 51 prior Nuss) [13]. Repair of patients with previous

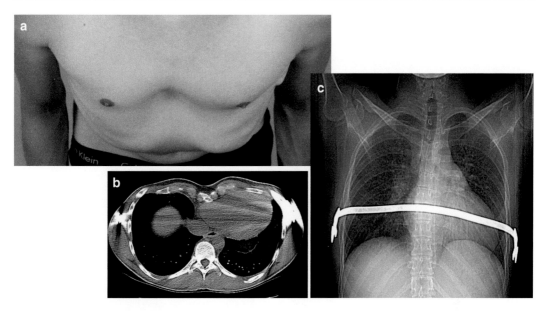

Fig. 15.8 (**a–c**) Photographs (**a**) and radiographic imaging (**b**, **c**) are shown of a 26 year-old male with pectus excavatum deformity 2 years after placement of single support bar with residual defect of Haller Index 4.6 and chronic postoperative pain. The single bar fails to elevate and support the defect inferiorly

Table 15.3 Frequent causes of failed or recurrent prior Ravitch/open procedures

Incomplete previous repair
Repair at too young of age
Dissection either too extensive or too little
Early removal or lack of support structures
Incomplete healing of the chest wall with pseudoarthrosis, "sternal floating and osteonecrosis"
Connective tissue disorders
Infection and seroma complications

Ravitch procedures required multiple bars. Opening the previous Ravitch incision for manual lifting of the sternum during the dissection under the pectus defect was felt to significantly improve the safety of the dissection and success of the procedure [13].

Rarely following Ravitch repair at too young and age, patients can have impairment of the normal chest wall growth, or acquired asphyxiating thoracic dystrophy, which was first described by Haller in 1996 [35]. Haller speculated that this "acquired Jeune's syndrome" was related to disruption of the normal growth centers of the affected ribs. These patients typically had repair of their defect at a very young age (<4 years), which had been common in the 1970s and 1980s. This is a complicated disorder with high risks for reconstruction to improve the chest defects presents. These patients required complex reconstructions of which discussion is beyond the context of this report and limited reports are published [21, 32, 35].

Indications for Surgical Revision Repair

Indications for repair of recurrent pectus excavatum are similar to those for primary repair and reviewed in Table 15.4 [1, 3–5, 9, 11, 14, 37, 64, 75–82]. Those patients with a recurrent, significant defect and those with symptomatology correlating with the return of their defect, including dyspnea, palpitations, and inability to keep up with their peers, all factor into the decision to repair a recurrent defect. Additionally, patients that have undergone previous open repair may have areas of non-union, chest wall hernias and other conditions that lead to chronic pain and chest wall instability [3, 33–35, 37, 71, 76].

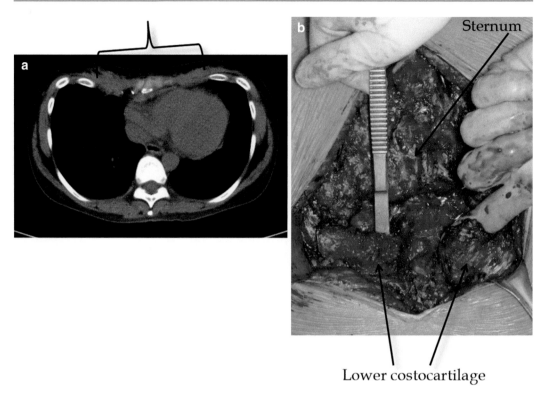

Fig. 15.9 (**a**, **b**) Computerized tomography (**a**) of the chest and intraoperative photograph (**b**) showing fibrous malunion and recurrence due to improper healing after prior Ravitch pectus repair. The instrument is place under the lower cartilage attachments which are completely separate from the sternum. *Arrows*

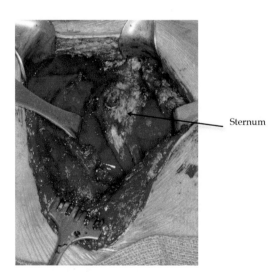

Fig. 15.10 Intraoperative photograph showing "sternal floating" after prior open Ravitch pectus repair with bilateral non-union of costocartilages and sternum

Resultant symptoms from this type of defect can be severe and may be an indication for surgery despite not meeting criteria based on the mea-

Table 15.4 Indications for surgical revision of prior failed pectus excavatum

Haller Index greater than 3.25 or Significant Correction Index
Continued evidence for Cardiac Compression
Symptomatology correlating with return of defect
Non-union, pseudoarthrosis or sternal/chest wall instability

surements of their defect. Reoperation should be individualized to the patient with great consideration given to the increased operative complexity and risk of complications. Extensive patient education about the surgical complications, recovery period, and final results are necessary to create realistic expectations for the patient.

In general, we have approached all our revision cases from a stepwise evaluation including:

1. **Physical exam** to identify areas of pseudoarthrosis and malunion between the sternum and ribs, or serial instability of the costal joints

"floating sternum" [36, 71]. Assessment of compliance and residual flexibility of anterior chest wall.

2. **CT or MRI** studies of the chest are necessary to allow for measurements of the defect, but also for visualization of areas of malunion or non-union that are not appreciated on physical exam. Identification of chest wall hernia, irregular cartilage regeneration at the retrosternal level and incomplete reunion of previous resection sites can be performed [70, 81, 83–85].

3. Evaluation of prior operative notes, chest roentgenograms and films relative to patient's prior procedures.

4. Evaluation of physiologic abnormalities which may include echocardiogram, pulmonary functions and cardiopulmonary V02 and exercise parameters [7, 23, 75, 80, 81, 86–92].

For the majority of reoperative patients, we plan MIRPE utilizing forced elevation (Johnson, ATS publication pending) (Fig. 15.11a, b). shows an algorithm for our approach to revision patients. Open resection with osteotomy and partial modified revision Ravitch are performed when necessary if the chest wall will not elevate adequately. Patients with pseudoarthrosis or "floating sternum" are planned for a combined procedure with elevation of the chest wall and stabilization of sternocostal instability [36, 71]. Patients with acquired thoracic dystrophy require more complex open reconstructions [32, 35] Table 15.5 outlines the operative steps:

Procedure Detailed Description

All patients are administered intravenous antibiotic prophylaxis prior to initiation of procedure. General anesthesia with double-lumen intubation is performed. A transesophageal echocardiogram probe is placed and cardiac compression, function, and absence of pericardial effusion documented throughout the case. The patient is placed in supine position with arms secured at the sides. Two longitudinal 5-in. rolls are placed under the back parallel to the spine and the arms padded and tucked at the sides. Groins are left exposed

and prepped into the surgical field should emergent access and cardiopulmonary bypass be necessary (Fig. 15.12). This positioning facilitates access to both anterior and lateral aspects of the chest wall for placing and affixing bars.

Single 3-cm incisions are made bilateral following the rib contour at the inferolateral pectoral borders. Incisions are positioned to allow access to the intercostal spaces adjacent to the defect. Submuscular pockets are developed utilizing electrocautery to elevate the pectoralis muscles off the chest wall along the anterior and lateral chest wall. Initially a 5 mm port is placed through the right incision and carbon dioxide insufflation to 5–8 mmHg pressure is utilized. A 5-mm flexible endoscope (Olympus 5-mm Endoeye Flex 5, Central Valley, PA) is placed and allows safe placement of a second 5 mm port inferiorly in the right chest for visualization of intrathoracic procedures. Careful takedown of intrathoracic adhesions is performed under direct visualization. No attempt to cross the mediastinum occurs until sternal elevation is achieved.

Elevation with the RulTract Retractor (Ruletract Inc., Cleveland, OH) is then attempted (Fig. 15.13) [55, 57].Two-mm incisions are placed on either side of the sternal defect and the perforating tips of a bone clamp (Lewin Spinal Perforating Forceps, V. Mueller NL6960; CareFusion, Inc, San Diego, CA) are inserted into the sternum. The clamp is then fully closed. The RuleTract Retractor is attached to the table at the level of the mid-sternum on the left side. The sternum is then attempted for elevation.

If Elevation Is Achieved, a Modified Nuss Will Be Performed for the Revision Case

Procedure for Modified Nuss for Revision

The first bar is positioned in the interspace at the superior aspect of the defect. A second bar is then placed 1–2 inner spaces below this one. If there is residual lower defect, a third bar will be placed (Fig. 15.14a, b). Bars are sized and shaped to best correct the patient's defect. We use shorter bar lengths and try to minimize the lateral extension of the bar around the chest. Bars are custom bent

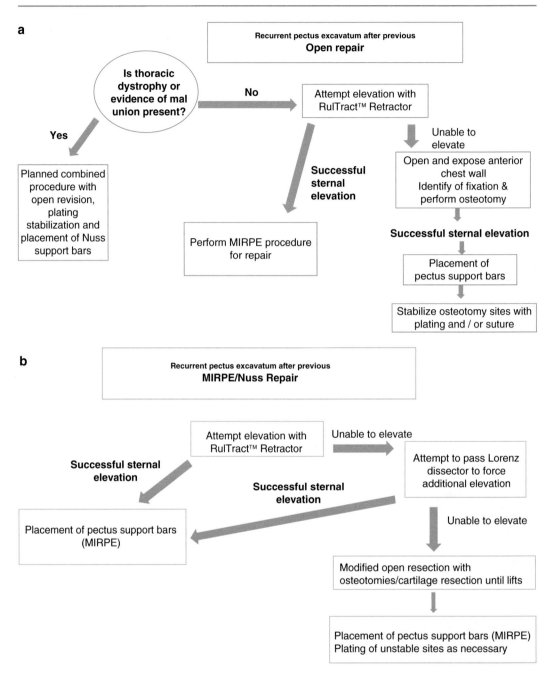

Fig. 15.11 (**a**, **b**) Algorithm for surgical approach to recurrent patients (**a**) previous Nuss/Minimally invasive pectus excavatum repair (**b**) open repair

and shaped for individual patients. Bars are flipped into place with the sternum still held elevated to minimize stress lateralized to the intercostal space. Bilateral circumferential fixation of the bars around the rib using FiberWire® (Arthrex

Inc, Naples, FL) is performed. The technique for this has been previously published [93]. Two or three sites of fixation are performed bilaterally for each bar. Fixation should incorporate the islet of the bar bilateral and incorporate a rib either

Table 15.5 Procedure for revision of prior Nuss and open PE recurrence

1. Attempt thoracoscopic MIRPE with forced sternal elevation with RulTract™
If able to achieve lift and no malunion, MIRPE is performed with adherence to principals of multiple, properly positioned, stabile bars for support
If unable to elevate successfully or evidence of malunion or sternal floating:
2. Prior open surgical incision is reopened or midline incision made and muscle flaps elevated to expose the anterior chest wall. Evaluation for sites of restriction to elevation are identified
3. Removal of deformed costal cartilages is performed at sites preventing elevation only. An anterior wedge osteotomy of the sternum and osteotomy cuts of fused sites are performed where required until anterior elevation of defect possible
4. Thoracoscopic placement of sternal support bars in 2–3 sites balancing defect is performed for MIRPE repair
5. Selective anterior stabilization of sternum, sternocostal nonunion and pseudoarthroses is performed utilizing titanium plating and FiberWire

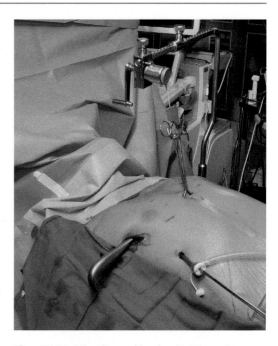

Fig. 15.13 Elevation with the RulTract Retractor (Ruletract Inc., Cleveland, OH) attached to the table at the level of the mid-sternum on the left side is attempted. A perforating tips bone clamp (Lewin Spinal Perforating Forceps, V. Mueller NL6960; CareFusion, Inc, San Diego, Calif) and attached to the retractor

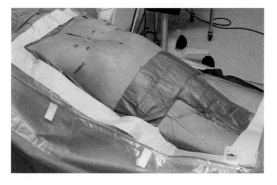

Fig. 15.12 All reoperative recurrent pectus excavatum patients are positioned supine with arms tucked at the sides and groins exposed should emergent cardiopulmonary bypass be necessary. This positioning facilitates access to both anterior and lateral aspects of the chest wall for placing and affixing bars

passing the right angle inferior to rib. The suture is then securely tied over the bar lying partly in the grooves.

If Forced Sternal Elevation Cannot Elevate the Chest Anteriorly or Malunion and Sternal Floating Evident

Procedure for Combined Open and Modified Nuss for Revision

If forced sternal elevation cannot elevate the chest anteriorly or malunion and sternal floating evident, the midline incision from patient's previous open procedure is excised and dissection taken down to the bony chest wall. Sites of calcified restriction or malunion are identified. If cartilage and perichondrium remains, a limited cartilage resection is performed. These techniques are similar to those used in the modified

directly below or on either side of the bar. A second and sometimes 3rd site of fixation should be placed more medial on each side closer to the rotational fulcrum depending on the pressure and stability of the bar placement. A small right angle is used to pass the FiberWire® suture through the intercostal space just above a rib and directed towards the apex. The suture is again grasped by

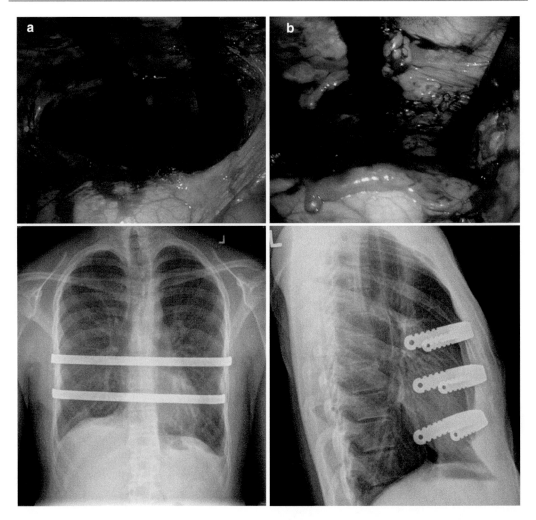

Fig. 15.14 (**a**, **b**) Intraoperative photograph and chest roentgenograms showing the placement of 2 and 3 Nuss support bars for repair of pectus excavatum deformity

Ravitch repairs, but are limited to areas that will not elevate and in sites with persistent malformation following elevation. For many patients, osteotomy of the sternum and improperly positioned, fused ribs may be required due to extensive scar tissue and calcification. In these scenarios, multiple osteotomies may be required at fixed sites and the sternochondral junctions using bone chisels or a powered bone saw.

Once chest mobility is obtained and anterior elevation is obtained with the RuleTract, exploration and takedown of the mediastinum is thoracoscopically performed. A combination of electrocautery and blunt dissection of pleural and

mediastinal adhesions is performed. In cases with significant pericardial adhesions to the sternum, a subxiphoid approach is additionally used for direct takedown of scar tissue by pulling the sternum upward and looking directly. Others have also reported using this approach to safely dissect thru the adherent mediastinal structures [5, 13, 31]. Once the dissection is complete, the Lorentz dissector (Biomet MicroFixation, Jacksonville, FL) is passed across from the right interspace to the contralateral side for guided placement of the support bars (Fig. 15.15). The procedure as previously described is performed for placement of 2–3 support bars and FiberWire securing.

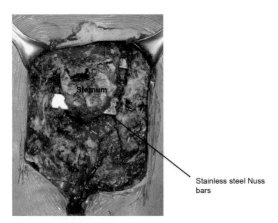

Fig. 15.15 Intraoperative photograph of patient with recurrent severe pectus excavatum after open Ravitch. Extensive malunion is seen. Areas of pseudoarthrosis and fibrous malunion are debrided back to healthy tissue. Stainless steel pectus bars are placed to elevate and support the chest anterior. Bone graft and plating will then be utilized to further stabilize and repair these sites

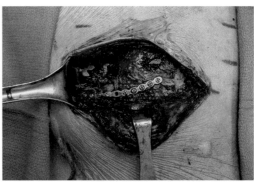

Fig. 15.16 Intraoperative photograph of titanium plating utilized to secure a site of malunion after failed Ravitch procedure

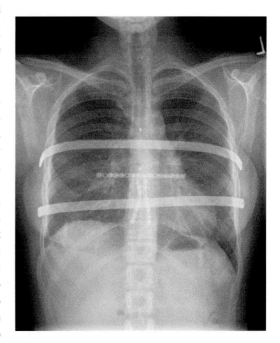

Fig. 15.17 Chest roentgenogram is shown of patient postoperative from revision procedure after recurrent Ravitch. Sites of malunion were stabilized with titanium plates. Two support Nuss bars were utilized

Extensive calcification of the chest wall following repair can be equally debilitating following open repair. Correction of this condition is extremely difficult, with the concern that any subsequent repair may result in a similar result as scarring occurs following operative intervention. Osteotomies of the sterno-costal junctions, as well as osteotomies more laterally along the ribs may be necessary to mobilize the anterior chest wall. Repeated osteotomies in similar locations are prone to malunion or non-union, which has led to our use of titanium plating or Fiberwire to stabilize these areas. Open repair can also lead to disruption of the blood supply to portions of the bony portions of the chest wall, which can lead to sections of the chest wall that are absent. These areas are difficult to stabilize, and titanium plating is at times necessary to restore chest wall stability [34, 37]. Titanium sternal plating (Biomet Microfixation, Jacksonville, FL and DePuy Synthes) and FiberWire fixation is then utilized to approximate the sites of costocartilage/rib to the sternum following elevation. Plates are chosen based on length and shape to best accommodate the fixation (Figs. 15.16 and 15.17). Multiple plates are utilized for all unstable areas and FiberWire for attachment to the sternum at other sites. For more extensive deformities with osteo- necrosis and extensive chest wall hernia, use of cadaveric bone graft, methylmethacrylate and biologic mesh can be utilized for repair. These more extensive techniques are covered in previous publications [32, 33].

Support bars are securely affixed to the chest wall and then the sternum is released and the bone clamp removed. The pectoralis muscles are reattached to the chest wall covering the bars and incisions closed with layered absorbable suture. A single approximating stitch is placed on the sites of the clamp insertion.

Once the chest wall defect is completely corrected, the pectoralis muscle and fascia, as well as the rectus abdominus muscle and fascia are reattached to the chest wall. The incisions are closed with layered absorbable suture. Chest tubes are placed through the lower port site on the right and left if deemed necessary.

Conclusion

Recurrence of pectus excavatum deformities occurs after both open and MIRPE. Recurrence risks are based on multiple factors and differ based on the initial repair procedure. Identifying the sources of a previous procedure's failure is critical to preventing the recurrence. Surgeon experience with the type of procedure is also important as reoperative cases can be difficult and are prone to increased complications. Complete correction of the pectus defect may not possible with MIRPE alone, and a combination of surgical techniques may be necessary in many patients. Each case must be taken on an individual basis based on that patient's anatomy and previous repair technique.

References

1. Ellis DG, Snyder CL, Mann CM. The 're-do' chest wall deformity correction. J Pediatr Surg. 1997;32(9):1267–71.
2. Antonoff MB, Erickson AE, Hess DJ, et al. When patients choose: comparison of Nuss, Ravitch, and Leonard procedures for primary repair of pectus excavatum. J Pediatr Surg. 2009;44(6):1113–8; discussion 118–9.
3. Colombani PM. Recurrent chest wall anomalies. Semin Pediatr Surg. 2003;12(2):94–9.
4. De Ugarte DA, Choi E, Fonkalsrud EW. Repair of recurrent pectus deformities. Am Surg. 2002;68(12):1075–9.
5. Guo L, Mei J, Ding F, et al. Modified Nuss procedure in the treatment of recurrent pectus excavatum after open repair. Interact Cardiovasc Thorac Surg. 2013;17(2):258–62.
6. Kelly RE, Goretsky MJ, Obermeyer R, et al. Twenty-one years of experience with minimally invasive repair of pectus excavatum by the Nuss procedure in 1215 patients. Ann Surg. 2010;252(6):1072–81.
7. Kelly Jr RE, Mellins RB, Shamberger RC, et al. Multicenter study of pectus excavatum, final report: complications, static/exercise pulmonary function, and anatomic outcomes. J Am Coll Surg. 2013;217(6):1080–9.
8. Liu T, Liu H, Li Y. Comparison of the Nuss and sternal turnover procedures for primary repair of pectus excavatum. Asian J Surg. 2014;37(1):30–4.
9. Luu TD, Kogon BE, Force SD, et al. Surgery for recurrent pectus deformities. Ann Thorac Surg. 2009;88(5):1627–31.
10. Mansour KA, Thourani VH, Odessey EA, et al. Thirty-year experience with repair of pectus deformities in adults. Ann Thorac Surg. 2003;76(2):391–5; discussion 395.
11. Miller KA, Ostlie DJ, Wade K, et al. Minimally invasive bar repair for 'redo' correction of pectus excavatum. J Pediatr Surg. 2002;37(7):1090–2.
12. Nasr A, Fecteau A, Wales PW. Comparison of the Nuss and the Ravitch procedure for pectus excavatum repair: a meta-analysis. J Pediatr Surg. 2010;45(5):880–6.
13. Redlinger Jr RE, Kelly Jr RE, Nuss D, et al. One hundred patients with recurrent pectus excavatum repaired via the minimally invasive Nuss technique-effective in most regardless of initial operative approach. J Pediatr Surg. 2011;46(6):1177–81.
14. Croitoru DP, Kelly Jr RE, Goretsky MJ, et al. The minimally invasive Nuss technique for recurrent or failed pectus excavatum repair in 50 patients. J Pediatr Surg. 2005;40(1):181–6; discussion 186–7.
15. Fonkalsrud EW. 912 open pectus excavatum repairs: changing trends, lessons learned: one surgeon's experience. World J Surg. 2009;33(2):180–90.
16. Willital GH, Meier H. Cause of funnel chest recurrences---operative treatment and long-term results. Prog Pediatr Surg. 1977;10:253–6.
17. Kasagi Y, Wada J, Nakajima H, et al. Re-operation of pectus excavatum. Nihon Kyobu Geka Gakkai Zasshi. 1989;37(3):540–5.
18. Aronson DC, Bosgraaf RP, van der Horst C, et al. Nuss procedure: pediatric surgical solution for adults with pectus excavatum. World J Surg. 2007;31(1):26–9; discussion 30.
19. Castellani C, Schalamon J, Saxena AK, et al. Early complications of the Nuss procedure for pectus excavatum: a prospective study. Pediatr Surg Int. 2008;24(6):659–66.
20. Croitoru DP, Kelly Jr RE, Goretsky MJ, et al. Experience and modification update for the minimally invasive Nuss technique for pectus excavatum repair in 303 patients. J Pediatr Surg. 2002;37(3):437–45.
21. Haller Jr JA. Complications of surgery for pectus excavatum. Chest Surg Clin N Am. 2000;10(2):415–26, ix.
22. Fonkalsrud EW, Reemtsen B. Force required to elevate the sternum of pectus excavatum patients. J Am Coll Surg. 2002;195:575–7.

23. Kelly Jr RE, Shamberger RC, Mellins RB, et al. Prospective multicenter study of surgical correction of pectus excavatum: design, perioperative complications, pain, and baseline pulmonary function facilitated by internet-based data collection. J Am Coll Surg. 2007;205(2):205–16.

24. Leonhardt J, Kubler JF, Feiter J, et al. Complications of the minimally invasive repair of pectus excavatum. J Pediatr Surg. 2005;40(11):e7–9.

25. Nuss D. Minimally invasive surgical repair of pectus excavatum. Semin Pediatr Surg. 2008;17(3):209–17.

26. Nuss D, Croitoru DP, Kelly Jr RE, et al. Review and discussion of the complications of minimally invasive pectus excavatum repair. Eur J Pediatr Surg. 2002; 12(4):230–4.

27. Park HJ, Chung WJ, Lee IS, et al. Mechanism of bar displacement and corresponding bar fixation techniques in minimally invasive repair of pectus excavatum. J Pediatr Surg. 2008;43(1):74–8.

28. Park HJ, Kim KS, Lee S, et al. A next-generation pectus excavatum repair technique: new devices make a difference. Ann Thorac Surg. 2015;99:455–61.

29. Arn PH, Scherer LR, Haller Jr JA, et al. Outcome of pectus excavatum in patients with Marfan syndrome and in the general population. J Pediatr. 1989;115(6): 954–8.

30. Vegunta RK, Pacheco PE, Wallace LJ, et al. Complications associated with the Nuss procedure: continued evolution of the learning curve. Am J Surg. 2008;195(3):313–6; discussion 316–7.

31. Liu JF, Zhu SH, Xu B. Early results of 18 adults, following a modified Nuss operation for recurrent pectus excavatum. Eur J Cardiothorac Surg. 2013;43(2):279–82.

32. Jaroszewski DE, Notrica DM, McMahon LE, et al. Operative management of acquired thoracic dystrophy in adults after open pectus excavatum repair. Ann Thorac Surg. 2014;97(5):1764–70.

33. Jaroszewski D, Johnson K, Lackey J, et al. Complex repair of pectus excavatum recurrence and massive chest wall defect and lung herniation after prior open repair. Ann Thorac Surg. 2013;96(2):e29–31.

34. Schulz-Drost S, Syed J, Besendoerfer M, et al. Elastic stable chest repair as a means of stabilizing the anterior chest wall in recurrent pectus excavatum with sternocostal pseudarthrosis: an innovative fixation device. Thorac Cardiovasc Surg. 2015;63:419–26.

35. Haller Jr JA, Colombani PM, Humphries CT, et al. Chest wall constriction after too extensive and too early operations for pectus excavatum. Ann Thorac Surg. 1996;61(6):1618–24; discussion 1625.

36. Prabhakaran K, Paidas CN, Haller JA, et al. Management of a floating sternum after repair of pectus excavatum. J Pediatr Surg. 2001;36(1):159–64.

37. Pasrija C, Wehman B, Singh DP, et al. Recurrent pectus excavatum repair via Ravitch technique with rib locking plates. Eplasty. 2014;14:ic46.

38. Cheng YL, Lee SC, Huang TW, et al. Efficacy and safety of modified bilateral thoracoscopy-assisted Nuss procedure in adult patients with pectus excavatum. Eur J Cardiothorac Surg. 2008;34(5):1057–61.

39. Coln D, Gunning T, Ramsay M, et al. Early experience with the Nuss minimally invasive correction of pectus excavatum in adults. World J Surg. 2002; 26(10):1217–21.

40. Hebra A, Jacobs JP, Feliz A, et al. Minimally invasive repair of pectus excavatum in adult patients. Am Surg. 2006;72(9):837–42.

41. Jaroszewski DE, Fonkalsrud EW. Repair of pectus chest deformities in 320 adult patients: 21 year experience. Ann Thorac Surg. 2007;84(2):429–33.

42. Johnson WR, Fedor D, Singhal S. Systematic review of surgical treatment techniques for adult and pediatric patients with pectus excavatum. J Cardiothorac Surg. 2014;9:25.

43. Park HJ, Sung SW, Park JK, et al. How early can we repair pectus excavatum: the earlier the better? Eur J Cardiothorac Surg. 2012;42(4):667–72.

44. Pilegaard HK, Licht PB. Routine use of minimally invasive surgery for pectus excavatum in adults. Ann Thorac Surg. 2008;86(3):952–6.

45. Ravenni G, Actis Dato GM, Zingarelli E, et al. Nuss procedure in adult pectus excavatum: a simple artifice to reduce sternal tension. Interact Cardiovasc Thorac Surg. 2013;17(1):23–5.

46. Schalamon J, Pokall S, Windhaber J, et al. Minimally invasive correction of pectus excavatum in adult patients. J Thorac Cardiovasc Surg. 2006;132(3):524–9.

47. Teh SH, Hanna AM, Pham TH, et al. Minimally invasive repair for pectus excavatum in adults. Ann Thorac Surg. 2008;85(6):1914–8.

48. Yoon YS, Kim HK, Choi YS, et al. A modified Nuss procedure for late adolescent and adult pectus excavatum. World J Surg. 2010;34(7):1475–80.

49. Wang L, Zhong H, Zhang FX, et al. Minimally invasive Nuss technique allows for repair of recurrent pectus excavatum following the Ravitch procedure: report of 12 cases. Surg Today. 2011;41(8):1156–60.

50. Hebra A, Swoveland B, Egbert M, et al. Outcome analysis of minimally invasive repair of pectus excavatum: review of 251 cases. J Pediatr Surg. 2000;35(2):252–7; discussion 257–8.

51. Huang PM, Wu ET, Tseng YT, et al. Modified Nuss operation for pectus excavatum: design for decreasing cardiopulmonary complications. Thorac Cardiovasc Surg. 2006;54(2):134–7.

52. Moss RL, Albanese CT, Reynolds M. Major complications after minimally invasive repair of pectus excavatum: case reports. J Pediatr Surg. 2001;36(1):155–8.

53. Nuss D, Kelly Jr RE, Croitoru DP, et al. A 10-year review of a minimally invasive technique for the correction of pectus excavatum. J Pediatr Surg. 1998; 33(4):545–52.

54. Park HJ. Technical innovations in the minimally invasive approach for treating pectus excavatum: a paradigm shift through six years' experience with 630 patients. Innovations (Phila). 2007;2(1):25–8.

55. Jaroszewski DE, Johnson K, McMahon L, et al. Sternal elevation before passing bars: a technique for improving visualization and facilitating minimally invasive pectus excavatum repair in adult patients. J Thorac Cardiovasc Surg. 2014;147(3):1093–5.

56. Weber PG, Huemmer HP, Reingruber B. Forces to be overcome in correction of pectus excavatum. J Thorac Cardiovasc Surg. 2006;132(6):1369–73.

57. Park HJ, Jeong JY, Jo WM, et al. Minimally invasive repair of pectus excavatum: a novel morphology-tailored, patient-specific approach. J Thorac Cardiovasc Surg. 2010;139(2):379–86.

58. Nagasao T, Miyamoto J, Tamaki T, et al. Stress distribution on the thorax after the Nuss procedure for pectus excavatum results in different patterns between adult and child patients. J Thorac Cardiovasc Surg. 2007;134(6):1502–7.

59. Pilegaard HK, Licht PB. Early results following the Nuss operation for pectus excavatum--a single-institution experience of 383 patients. Interact Cardiovasc Thorac Surg. 2008;7(1):54–7.

60. Papandria D, Arlikar J, Sacco Casamassima MG, et al. Increasing age at time of pectus excavatum repair in children: emerging consensus? J Pediatr Surg. 2013;48(1):191–6.

61. Olbrecht VA, Arnold MA, Nabaweesi R, et al. Lorenz bar repair of pectus excavatum in the adult population: should it be done? Ann Thorac Surg. 2008; 86(2):402–8; discussion 408–9.

62. Pilegaard HK. Extending the use of Nuss procedure in patients older than 30 years. Eur J Cardiothorac Surg. 2011;40(2):334–7.

63. Lodge AJ, Wells WJ, Backer CL, et al. A novel bioresorbable film reduces postoperative adhesions after infant cardiac surgery. Ann Thorac Surg. 2008;86(2): 614–21.

64. Pison CJ, Gonzalez AG, Perez MA, et al. Correction of recurrent pectus excavatum post-Ravitch with the Nuss technique. Cir Pediatr. 2009;22(2):77–80.

65. Ravitch MM. The operative treatment of pectus excavatum. Ann Surg. 1949;129(4):429–44.

66. Ravitch MM. New trends in pediatric surgery; pectus excavatum, esophageal atresia, intussusception, Hirschsprung's disease. Surg Clin North Am. 1949; 29(4):1535–50.

67. Fonkalsrud EW, Anselmo DM. Less extensive techniques for repair of pectus carinatum: the undertreated chest deformity. J Am Coll Surg. 2004;198(6): 898–905.

68. Davis JT, Weinstein S. Repair of the pectus deformity: results of the Ravitch approach in the current era. Ann Thorac Surg. 2004;78(2):421–6.

69. Robicsek F, Watts LT, Fokin AA. Surgical repair of pectus excavatum and carinatum. Semin Thorac Cardiovasc Surg. 2009;21(1):64–75.

70. Chang PY, Lai JY, Chen JC, et al. Quantitative evaluation of bone and cartilage changes after the Ravitch thoracoplasty by multislice computed tomography with 3-dimensional reconstruction. J Thorac Cardiovasc Surg. 2007;134(5):1279–83.

71. Renz J, Reyes C. Repair of a floating sternum with autologous rib grafts and polylactide bioabsorbable struts in an 18-year-old male. J Pediatr Surg. 2012;47(12):e27–30.

72. Johnson WR, Fedor D, Singhal S. A novel approach to eliminate cardiac perforation in the nuss procedure. Ann Thorac Surg. 2013;95(3):1109–11.

73. Takagi S, Oyama T, Tomokazu N, et al. A new sternum elevator reduces severe complications during minimally invasive repair of the pectus excavatum. Pediatr Surg Int. 2012;28(6):623–6.

74. Belcher E, Arora S, Samancilar O, et al. Reducing cardiac injury during minimally invasive repair of pectus excavatum. Eur J Cardiothorac Surg. 2008; 33(5):931–3.

75. Colombani PM. Preoperative assessment of chest wall deformities. Semin Thorac Cardiovasc Surg. 2009; 21(1):58–63.

76. Kelly Jr RE. Pectus excavatum: historical background, clinical picture, preoperative evaluation and criteria for operation. Semin Pediatr Surg. 2008;17(3):181–93.

77. Kragten HA, Siebenga J, Hoppener PF, et al. Symptomatic pectus excavatum in seniors (SPES): a cardiovascular problem? : A prospective cardiological study of 42 senior patients with a symptomatic pectus excavatum. Neth Heart J. 2011;19(2):73–8.

78. Krasopoulos G, Dusmet M, Ladas G, et al. Nuss procedure improves the quality of life in young male adults with pectus excavatum deformity. Eur J Cardiothorac Surg. 2006;29(1):1–5.

79. Lester CW. The surgical treatment of funnel chest. Ann Surg. 1946;123(6):1003–22.

80. Maagaard M, Tang M, Ringgaard S, et al. Normalized cardiopulmonary exercise function in patients with pectus excavatum three years after operation. Ann Thorac Surg. 2013;96(1):272–8.

81. Swanson JW, Avansino JR, Phillips GS, et al. Correlating Haller Index and cardiopulmonary disease in pectus excavatum. Am J Surg. 2012;203(5):660–4.

82. Jaroszewski D, Notrica D, McMahon L, et al. Current management of pectus excavatum: a review and update of therapy and treatment recommendations. J Am Board Fam Med. 2010;23(2):230–9.

83. Coln E, Carrasco J, Coln D. Demonstrating relief of cardiac compression with the Nuss minimally invasive repair for pectus excavatum. J Pediatr Surg. 2006;41(4):683–6; discussion 683–6.

84. Goretsky MJ, Kelly Jr RE, Croitoru D, et al. Chest wall anomalies: pectus excavatum and pectus carinatum. Adolesc Med Clin. 2004;15(3):455–71.

85. Haller Jr JA, Kramer SS, Lietman SA. Use of CT scans in selection of patients for pectus excavatum surgery: a preliminary report. J Pediatr Surg. 1987;22(10):904–6.

86. Gahrton G. ECG changes in pectus excavatum (funnel chest). A pre- and postoperative study. Acta Med Scand. 1961;170:431–8.

87. Krueger T, Chassot PG, Christodoulou M, et al. Cardiac function assessed by transesophageal echocardiography during pectus excavatum repair. Ann Thorac Surg. 2010;89(1):240–3.

88. Maagaard M, Udholm S, Hjortdal VE, et al. Right ventricular outflow tract obstruction caused by a displaced pectus bar 30 months following the Nuss procedure. Eur J Cardiothorac Surg. 2015;47:e42–3.

89. Malek MH, Berger DE, Housh TJ, et al. Cardiovascular function following surgical repair of pectus excavatum: a metaanalysis. Chest. 2006;130(2):506–16.

90. Malek MH, Coburn JW. Strategies for cardiopulmonary exercise testing of pectus excavatum patients. Clinics (Sao Paulo). 2008;63(2):245–54.

91. Neviere R, Wurtz A. Longer term effects of closed repair of pectus excavatum on cardiopulmonary status. J Pediatr Surg. 2013;48(9):1988–9.

92. Tang M, Nielsen HH, Lesbo M, et al. Improved cardiopulmonary exercise function after modified Nuss operation for pectus excavatum. Eur J Cardiothorac Surg. 2012;41(5):1063–7.

93. McMahon LE, Johnson KN, Jaroszewski DE, et al. Experience with FiberWire for pectus bar attachment. J Pediatr Surg. 2014;49(8):1259–63.

Role of Plastic Surgery in Chest Wall Corrections

16

Simon Withey and Robert A. Pearl

Abstract

Adjustment and augmentation of the soft tissues plays an important role in the management of patients with chest wall deformities. Both patients with severe abnormalities that have undergone reconstructive surgery to re-shape the chest wall and those with milder deformities can benefit from such soft tissue augmentation. This chapter discusses a range of autologous and/or implant based techniques that can be useful in these patients to provide an optimum result. The challenges of managing breast asymmetry or hypoplasia in the female patient with a chest wall deformity is also discussed.

Keywords

Chest wall deformities • Implants • Mammoplasty • Fat grafting

This section will cover surgery to augment the soft tissues of the chest to disguise chest wall deformities. Some patients may require reconstructive surgery to re-shape the chest wall either for functional or aesthetic reasons, but many will benefit from simpler surgery designed to disguise, rather than correct, the deformity. It is worth stressing that the patient's and the surgeon's perception of deformity can often be quite different, and, what the surgeon may consider quite minor adjustments to the soft tissues, relative to thoracic wall surgery, can make a huge difference to the patient.

Pectus excavatum, pectus carinatum and Poland's syndrome are the commonest abnormalities that require augmentation. In female patients varying degrees of breast hypoplasia and/or asymmetry often co-exist with the chest wall deformity that adds an extra complexity.

S. Withey, MBBS, FRCS FRCS(Ed) FRCS(Plast) (✉)
Department of Plastic and Reconstructive Surgery,
The Royal Free Hospital,
University College Hospital London,
London, UK
e-mail: simon.withey@mac.com

R.A. Pearl, MD, FRCS(Plast)
Department of Plastic and Reconstructive Surgery,
Queen Victoria Hospital, East Grinstead, UK

Clinical Assessment

We believe that it is very helpful if patients with chest wall deformities are seen in a combined Thoracic/Plastic Surgery clinic. A full history

© Springer International Publishing Switzerland 2016
S.K. Kolvekar, H.K. Pilegaard (eds.), *Chest Wall Deformities and Corrective Procedures*,
DOI 10.1007/978-3-319-23968-2_16

should be taken with particular emphasis on exercise tolerance and symptoms such as chest pain, palpitations or dizziness on exertion. The patient's attitude towards their deformity and motivations behind seeking treatment should also be discussed and carefully considered. It is critical that the expectations of surgery are considered in detail. Chest wall deformities can produce significant psychological trauma and dysmorphia and this is often the prime motivating factor for patients to seek corrective surgery, regardless of symptoms. Some may have unrealistic expectations of what can be achieved with surgery and involvement of a clinical psychologist is often advisable, both to help with the decision making process and also in preparation for any augmentation surgery. Female patients with pectus excavatum or Poland's syndrome also commonly have a degree of breast hypoplasia or asymmetry, and it may be this that is their primary concern. Women requesting breast augmentation with chest wall deformities, which, if mild, may have gone unnoticed by the patient, must be carefully examined and counseled. Studies have suggested almost 10 % of patients presenting with breast asymmetry have an underlying chest wall deformity [1]. Breast augmentation without addressing the underlying chest wall problem often magnifies the deformity and produces an unsatisfactory aesthetic appearance. The young female patient with chest wall abnormalities also merits special consideration, as future growth and breast development must be factored in to any treatment plan.

A full general examination should be then performed but with particular attention paid to general thoracic appearance and the cardiovascular system.

The degree and depth of the chest wall deformity should be noted and measured, and clinical photographs must be obtained. Evidence of sternal rotation, asymmetry and angulation should be recorded as should any spinal abnormalities such as kyphosis or scoliosis. In addition, features of connective tissue disorders (e.g. Marfan's, Ehlers Danlos, Noonan's) must be specifically looked for. The absence of the sternal head of pectoralis major is diagnostic for Poland's syndrome, although a range of unilateral chest wall and upper limb anomalies may be present. Syndactyly and symbrachydactyly are the commonest congenital hand deformities seen in Poland's syndrome, and whilst surgery for these is normally performed in early childhood, any planned future interventions need to be factored in to the management plan. In female patients full breast examination should be performed, and, in particular, any asymmetry noted.

Investigations

Investigations are dictated to some degree by the clinical findings, but patients with marked chest wall deformities, e.g. pectus excavatum, should have the following routinely performed.

Chest CT and 3D reconstruction This will give the *Haller index* (maximal transverse diameter/narrowest AP length of chest), which measures the degree of pectus excavatum.

Electrocardiogram and Echocardiogram These will assess whether deformity is affecting cardiac function. Furthermore, in Marfan's syndrome, it is important to check the aortic root is not aneurysmal.

Lung function tests This will provide not only measurements of vital capacity but also identify and restrictive or obstructive patterns of pulmonary dysfunction.

The majority of these investigations will guide the surgeon to the need for functional corrective surgery.

Clinical photographs are essential both for surgical planning and to document pre and post-operative appearances.

Treatment

The indications and type of surgery performed will depend on a range of physiological and psychological factors. Surgical treatment for chest wall deformities can be broadly split into procedures that camouflage, or those that re-shape and reconstruct, the thoracic cage. The latter is normally indicated in patients with evidence of physiological compromise, or for those with deformities so pronounced that camouflaging procedures alone with not be adequate. The modified Radvitch procedure or the Nuss procedures are the two common operations performed by Plastic or Thoracic surgeons to re-shape the chest wall. However, some patients will have defects that do not warrant such extensive surgery, some will decline it, and some, having undergone reshaping of the thoracic cage, will require further soft tissue adjustments to obtain final aesthetic result that both patient and surgeon are happy with.

Surgery to achieve augmentation of the soft tissues to disguise the bony deformity of the chest/sternum may involve the use of, autograft, such as autologous fat transfer, or synthetic implants, e.g. custom made silicone prosthesis. In female patients, concomitant breast hypoplasia made need to be addressed.

Custom Made Silicone Prostheses

Insertion of a custom-made silicone prostheses is a useful technique to camouflage chest wall deformities when thoracic cage surgery is not indicated, or is declined. Pectus excavatum in slim females is particularly conspicuous, and the resultant slope of the breast base causes the breast to "disappear" into the thoracic concavity extenuating any breast asymmetry or hypoplasia.

In these female patients the presence of breast tissue in the sternal concavity makes traditional "bedside" moulage techniques inaccurate for pre-operative planning and three-dimensional imaging with CT or MRI is increasingly used for creating accurate templates. A moulage or a template is used to provide an accurate representation of the defect on which the prosthesis may be modeled. It is advisable that the prosthetist and surgeon meet the patient together to carefully consider the surface area and depth of the defect, the thickness of the soft tissues overlying the contour defect and the patient's priorities and expectations. The mass of a prosthesis, its stiffness, and the position and thickness of its margins are the main determinants of implant palpability and visibility. Great efforts should be taken during planning to affect the implant design to avoid a conspicuous edge. Thin implant edges should be avoided where the soft tissues are particularly thin, as these are easily distorted if created at the lower margin as silicone buckles and bends under the weight of the prosthesis. The mass of the implant can be reduced by removing cores from the central segment.

Chest wall prostheses are normally inserted via a subcostal incision and a right-angled lighted retractor allows large pockets to be dissected with incisions of about 5 cm. It is important to obtain full haemostasis and the use of drains is advised.

The disadvantages are common to any prosthetic implant, and include infection, displacement and capsular contracture. Seromas are common, and may require repeated aspiration if large. As described earlier, implant palpability and visibility and "ghosting" are common features especially in slim patients. Patients should be advised to expect such occurrences.

Implant Mammoplasty

Breast hypoplasia and/or asymmetry often co-exist with chest wall deformities, and both abnormalities should be taken into account when planning surgery of the chest wall. Furthermore, it is not uncommon to see patients complaining of their breast appearance, who, when examined, are found to have normal breasts but a distorted chest wall. A normal breast tilted into the concavity of a pectus deformity will appear smaller than its true volume, and, asymmetry that is frequently found in patients with pectus deformities may be exaggerated if the breasts sit at a different angle and the breast base is at a different height.

For the best aesthetic results female patients with breast hypoplasia associated with a pronounced chest wall deformity should have surgical re-shaping of the thoracic cage before implant mammoplasty. Excellent results can be obtained in these patients [2].

For chest wall deformities that do not warrant thoracic surgery, the decision-making is less clear-cut. Suggestions that manubriosternal prominence can sometimes be camouflaged by slightly higher and more medially placed implants overlook the other implications of such surgery. Excessively medialised implants will introduce palpability, and in the longer term, rippling and wrinkling and we have seen several cases of symmastia when overenthusiastic attempts have been made to medialise breast implants in order to hide a pectus defect and these deformities are extremely difficult to correct. In pectus excavatum, it has been suggested that once the depth of the concavity is greater than 4 cm, or the width greater than 8 cm breast, implants alone will produce too deep or flat a cleavage [3]. In such cases, if thoracic reconstruction is not proposed, custom-made silicone prosthesis may be inserted to correct the chest wall first, before implant mammoplasty is considered. In many patients, "correction" of the chest wall deformity, whether by thoracic reshaping or insertion of a custom-made prosthesis may be all that is required. Providing a flat, stable base for the breast may resolve an apparent breast asymmetry or hypoplasia, which was merely a result of one or both of the breasts 'falling' into the sternal concavity.

The placement of breast implants will be dictated to some extent by the state of the chest wall musculature and specifically the medial origin of the pectoralis major which, in cases of pectus excavatum, is often more lateral than normal.

In female patients with pectus carinatum, augmentation mammoplasty may exaggerate or disguise the abnormality. The position and the extent of the deformity and the angulation of the breast base, the breast volume and width must be assessed carefully before a decision to operate is taken. Given the almost infinite varieties of combined deformities and breast morphology it is almost impossible to provide an algorithm to help in these cases, but in our experience, if the surgeon is reasonably experienced and takes the time to consider whether an implant might accentuate the deformity, it is usually fairly easy to make some prediction of outcome.

Autologous Fat Transfer

Autologous fat is widely used as a natural filler in plastic surgery for both reconstructive and aesthetic purposes. It is used commonly in the face and increasingly in the breast, both for both reconstruction and primary augmentation. The use of fat grafting to restore contour in patients with chest wall deformities is less widely reported, though we have found it a useful technique for patients with mild to moderate pectus excavatum, or in combination with the Nuss, or the modified Radvitch, procedure in more severe cases.

Fat transfer is a simple, low risk technique that can be performed as day case surgery. The fat is harvested via a specific fat harvesting cannula from an area of excess, it is centrifuged to separate the adipose cells (Fig. 16.1) which are then sequentially injected in small aliquots into the defect The introduction of many aliquots of small volume, into multiple tissue planes, maximizes the opportunity for revascularization and reduces the risk of lumpiness and irregularities. Integrated systems, such as the *Cytori PureGraft*™, are now available which will harvest, separate and purify the adipose cells ready for injection, removing the need for centrifugation. Such techniques allow the preparation of larger volumes of fat in a much less time consuming manner compared to traditional techniques. This is useful in chest wall defects where, in our experience it is not unusual to use at least 200 ml of injected fat to camouflage a defect. Figures 16.2 and 16.3 demonstrate pre and post-operative appearances of pectus excavatum treated with autologous fat grafting.

Once the transferred fat has been revascularised it may be viewed a permanent filler. However, autologous fat transfer is invariably associated with some early resorption of transferred fat, and a degree of "over augmentation" is advised. Despite this, it is likely that repeated procedures will be required. The complications of fat grafting, including fat necrosis, cyst formation and calcification are well recognized and rarely cause significant morbidity. Transferred fat cells will be subject to hypertrophy and atrophy as body weight changes. The major advantage of fat grating is than it removes any longer

Fig. 16.1 Harvested fat is separated by standard techniques before transfer

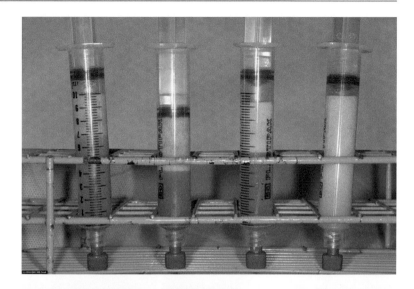

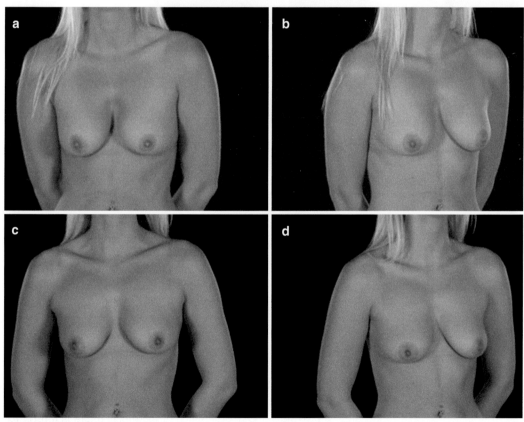

Fig. 16.2 Mild pectus excavatum in a female patient pre-operatively (**a**, **b**), and following fat grafting (**c**, **d**)

term implant related problems. The presence of adipose derived mesenchymal stem cells (ADMSC) within the transferred fat, play an adipogenic and angiogenic role, are thought to be largely responsible for graft survival and stem cell enriched fat grafts have become increasingly used. Transferred fat has had reportedly positive restorative effects on surrounding soft tissues, particularly in previously irradiated areas or heavily scarred chronic wounds.

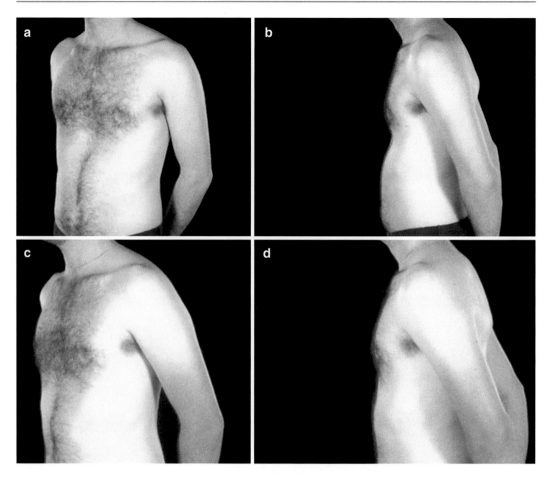

Fig. 16.3 Mild pectus excavatum in a male patient pre-operatively (**a**, **b**), and following fat grafting (**c**, **d**)

Flap Transfer

Given the relative successes of the aforementioned techniques flap reconstruction is less commonly used in these cases. An occasional exception is Poland's syndrome. Bipolar transfer of the latissimus dorsi muscle (LD) can reconstruct the anterior axillary fold and provide some bulk to replace the absent pectoralis major in these patients. The LD is raised as a muscle flap and rotated on its thoracodorsal pedicle to the front of the chest. The key step to provide a satisfactory contour of the anterior axillary fold involves detaching the LD from its humeral insertion and reattaching on the bicipital groove anterior to the neurovascular bundle. Although this transfer has been described as a functional reconstruction for the absent (or hypoplastic) pectoralis major, it is primarily used for aesthetic purposes. The LD muscle can also be affected in Poland's syndrome and its presence and bulk should be confirmed clinically prior to planning any surgery.

Flap transfer of all, or part, of the greater omentum has also been reported, normally in combination with a prosthesis, for chest wall reconstruction in Poland's syndrome with satisfactory results [4, 5]. Laparoscopic techniques enabling flap harvest without need for laparotomy. Our experience of the omental flap is mostly for reconstruction following sternal wound dehiscence post midline sternotomy, and we have found it a useful and reliable flap in this situation. However, the omental flap's versatility and ability to contour, suggest it may well have a role in selected cases of chest wall deformity.

Conclusions

Over the past 20 years an increasing emphasis on body image and shape has led to more patients with chest wall deformities to present to the Plastic Surgeon seeking corrective surgery. These deformities will range in severity and it is not always necessary to reconstruct the thoracic cage to obtain a good aesthetic result. Simpler, augmentation surgery such as autologous fat grafting and use of custom made silicone prostheses can often produce the desired result. Moreover, these techniques can be useful for to improve or refine the appearance of chest walls that have previously undergone reconstruction and reshaping of the thoracic cage. For patients presenting with significant distress over what appear to be minor deformities, surgeons should be aware of the diagnosis of body dysmorphic disorder, an under-diagnosed condition, and enlist the help of a clinical psychologist where appropriate.

References

1. Rohrich RJ, Hartley W, Brown S. Incidence of breast and chest wall asymmetry in breast augmentation: a retrospective analysis of 100 patients. Plast Reconstr Surg. 2006;118(7 Suppl):7S–13.
2. Bodin F, Bruant-Rodier C, Wilk A, Wihim JM. Surgical correction of pectus excavatum deformity and hypomastia. Eur J Plast Surg. 2008;31:15–20.
3. Hodgkinson D. Management of anterior chest wall deformity in breast augmentation. In: Shiffman M, editor. Breast augmentation. Berlin: Springer Publishing; 2009. p. 333–43.
4. Romanini MV, Vidal C, Godoy J, Morovic CG. Laparoscopically harvested omental flap for breast reconstruction in Poland's syndrome. J Plast Reconstr Aesthet Surg. 2013;66(11):e303–9.
5. dos Santos Costa S, Blotta RM, Mariano MB, Meurer L, Edelweiss MI. Aesthetic improvements in Poland's syndrome treatment with omentum flap. Aesthetic Plast Surg. 2010;34(5):634–9.

Non-surgical Treatment for Pectus Excavatum and Carinatum

Frank-Martin Haecker and Marcelo Martinez-Ferro

Abstract

Pectus excavatum (PE) and carinatum (PC) are characterized by an abnormal overgrowth of sternal and costal cartilages, which result in a depression or protrusion of the sternum and costal cartilages, respectively. Both chest wall malformations are cosmetic and functional pathologies. Whereas PE is commonly associated to cardiopulmonary dysfunction, PC causes deformation of the entire thoracic cage. PE is generally corrected operatively. In contrast, due to inherent risks of a major surgery, only severe cases of PC are operated. One of the authors (FMH) will describe his 12 years experience with vacuum bells to treat PE patients conservatively. The use of vacuum bells allow significant lift of the ribs and sternum, until definitive correction of cartilage growth takes place. When employed during minimally invasive repair of PE (MIRPE), vacuum bells can also be used as a tool to enhance retrosternal dissection, advancement of the pectus introducer and insertion and flipping of the pectus bar/s. The other author (MMF) will describe his 13 years experience with the FMF® Dynamic Compressor System to treat patients with PC conservatively. When considering results, there should be little doubt that no patient would be selected as a candidate for surgery before trying a non-operative approach. Further evaluation and follow-up studies are still necessary for both conservative approaches, though.

F.-M. Haecker, MD, FEAPU (✉)
Department of Pediatric Surgery,
University Children's Hospital, Basel, Switzerland
e-mail: frankmartin.haecker@ukbb.ch

M. Martinez-Ferro, MD
Department of Surgery,
Fundacion Hospitalaria Children's Hospital,
Buenos Aires, Argentina

© Springer International Publishing Switzerland 2016
S.K. Kolvekar, H.K. Pilegaard (eds.), *Chest Wall Deformities and Corrective Procedures*,
DOI 10.1007/978-3-319-23968-2_17

Keywords

Pectus excavatum • Pectus carinatum • Conservative treatment • Non-operative treatment • Vacuum bell • Dynamic Compressor System

Introduction

Pectus Excavatum (PE) and Carinatum (PC) are characterized by an abnormal overgrowth of sternal and costal cartilages, which result in a depression or protrusion of the sternum and costal cartilages, respectively.

Far from being an aesthetical condition, patients not only manifest psychological problems and disorders (discomfort, shame, shyness, anxiety, anguish, depression and social isolation), but also a series of physical signs and symptoms as chondrosternal and/or chondrocostal pain, sport intolerance, scoliosis, posterior asymmetry, impaired shoulders, kyphotic position, and specially in the case of PE patients, history of bronchospasms, repeated and prolonged respiratory disease, diminished stroke volume and mild to moderate heart dysfunction (in general only revealed by an echo stress test or cardiac MRI; not by usual exams). Cardio-respiratory disorders are very rare in PC patients, yet progressive thoracic cage deformation becomes evident with age.

PE is, in general, treated operatively, namely by Ravitch and variations, Nuss=Minimally Invasive Repair of Pectus Excavatum (MIRPE) or other techniques [1–8]. Among these variants, the authors prefer to operate on patients using the Nuss technique (MIRPE), described in 1998 by Dr. Donald Nuss et al. [9].

Consequent to the intrinsic risks of a major surgery, the operative treatment for PC was reserved for the most severe cases. Many PC patients remained untreated as a result.

Along the course of time, different non-operative approaches have been proposed to deal with these untreated PC patients [10–16]. One of the authors (MMF) co-invented with his partner, Dr. Carlos Fraire, the FMF® Dynamic Compressor System (DCS), and will hereby describe his 13 years experience with it [17–19].

On the other hand, the non-operative approach for PE, first published by Schier et al. consists in the utilization of vacuum bells in selected cases. The other author (FMH) will give an account of his 12 years experience with vacuum bells to treat PE patients non-operatively as well as during MIRPE [20–22].

Pectus Excavatum

Introduction

During last century, surgical repair represented the gold standard to correct PE in childhood and adolescents as well as adult patients. Previously used operative techniques to correct PE were largely based on open procedures and minimally invasive techniques. In 1998, Nuss et al. reported for the first time, their 10-year experience using a new technique of minimally invasive repair of PE (MIRPE) [9]. Today, the MIRPE technique is well established and represents a commonly used technique [23–26]. However, with its widespread use, the character and number of complications has increased [23–25, 27, 28]. Moreover, numerous recent studies report on an increasing number of near fatal complications [28–34]. Furthermore, in many cases of PE, the degree of pectus deformity does not immediately warrant surgery. Some patients are reluctant to undergo surgery because of the pain associated with the postoperative recovery and the risk of imperfect results.

In this situation, the introduction of the vacuum bell for conservative treatment of PE has made this alternative therapy a focus of interest for patients and physicians. The procedure of applying a vacuum to elevate the sternum was first used more than 100 years ago [35]. Spitzy and Lange reported their experience using a glass bell to correct PE [36]. Inadequate material and relevant side effects eliminated the routine use of this method for conservative treatment of PE. Despite the above-mentioned risks and unsatisfactory results after operative therapy for some patients, there has been little progress in the therapeutic use of the vacuum therapy during the last few decades. In the meantime, materials have improved and the vacuum devices can now exert strong forces. In 1992, the engineer Klobe E, who himself suffered from a PE, developed a special device for conservative treatment of PE [37]. Using his device during a period of 2.5 years, he was able to elevate the sternum and to correct his funnel chest to an extent that no funnel was visible any more [37].

Preliminary results from pilot studies using this method proved to be promising [20, 21]. Information on such new therapeutic modalities circulates not only among surgeons and paediatricians, but also rapidly among patients. In particular patients who refused operative treatment by previously available procedures, now appear at the outpatient clinic and request to be considered for this method.

The Vacuum Bell

Description
A suction cup is used to create a vacuum at the chest wall. The body of the vacuum bell is made of a silicon ring and a transparent polycarbonate window. A vacuum up to 15 % below atmospheric pressure is created by the patient using a hand pump (Fig. 17.1). Three different sizes (16 cm, 19 cm and 26 cm in diameter) exist allowing selection according to the individual patients age and shape of the ventral body surface (Fig. 17.2). The medium size model is available in a supplemental version with a reinforced silicon wall (type "bodybuilder"), e.g. for adult patients with a small deep PE. Additionally, a model fitted for young girls and women is available (Fig. 17.3). Pilot studies performed by Schier and Bahr [20] showed that the device lifted the sternum and ribs immediately. We could also confirm this effect by thoracoscopy during the MIRPE procedure [22]. According to the user instructions and our

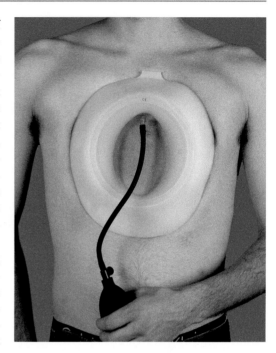

Fig. 17.1 Application of the vacuum bell

experience, the vacuum bell should be used for a minimum of 30 min, twice per day, and may be used up to a maximum of several hours daily. The vacuum bells by E. Klobe are CE certified and patent registered. In USA, the device was approved by the food and drug administration (FDA) in May 2012.

Indication and Contraindication
Indication for conservative therapy with the vacuum bell include patients who present with mild degree of PE and/or who want to avoid surgical procedure. In particular patients under the age of 10 years with a still flexible and elastic chest wall represent good candidates to start with the application.

Contraindications of the method comprise skeletal disorders, vasculopathies, coagulopathies and cardiac disorders [38]. To exclude these disorders, a standardised evaluation protocol was routinely performed before beginning the therapy.

Complications and relevant side effects include subcutaneous hematoma, petechial bleeding, dorsalgia and transient paresthesia of the upper extremities during the application.

Fig. 17.2 Vacuum bell in three different sizes (left 16 cm, middle 19 cm, right 26 cm in diameter)

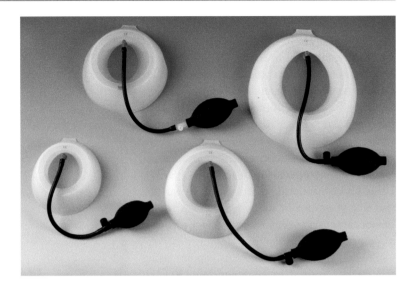

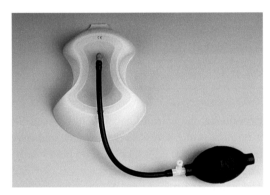

Fig. 17.3 Vacuum bell, model for adolescent girls/women

Methodology

All patients who visit our specialized outpatient clinic for chest wall deformities are informed about the option of conservative vs. surgical therapy to correct PE. Standardised evaluation includes history of the patient and his family, clinical examination and photo documentation of the PE. The depth of PE is measured in a standardized supine position. When the patient and/or the parents decide to perform the conservative vacuum therapy, meticulous family history is necessary to capture the above-mentioned contraindications. To exclude cardiac anomalies, we do routinely cardiac evaluation with electrocardiogram and echocardiography before starting the daily application in every patient.

Conservative Treatment

The first application of the vacuum bell occurs during the outpatient clinic visit under supervision of the attending physician. The appropriate size and model of the different type is defined. Patients learn the proper application of the device. In children under the age of 10 years, parents are instructed to use the device and children apply the vacuum bell under supervision of their parents or caregivers, respectively. The middle of the window should be positioned above the deepest point of the PE. Starting the application, the hand pump should be activated with 2–3 pumps. Patients are usually in a supine position for the first application. During therapy, most adolescent and adult patients apply the device in an upright position whereas parents of children under the age of 10 years prefer to continue in a supine position. With the device in position, patients may move and walk around in their home environment.

In patients with a localized deformity, it could be helpful to apply the device using the small model. In patients with an asymmetric PE or a grand canyon type PE, it could be useful to apply the device in changing positions.

When cardiac anomalies and other contraindications are excluded, patients may start with the daily application. All users are recommended to start to use the device twice daily for 30 min each. During follow-up, some patients follow the user instructions applying the device twice daily for 30 min each. However, some of the adult patients use the vacuum bell up to 8 h daily during office hours. A group of adolescent boys apply the device every night for 7–8 h. Since there does not yet exist a detailed study protocol for the application, the duration and frequency of daily application depends on the patients' individual decision and motivation.

Patients undergo follow-up at 3–6 monthly intervals including clinical examination, measurement of depth of PE and photo documentation. Clinical examination focuses on the improvement of depth of PE as well as on relevant side effects such as persistent hematoma and/or skin irritation. If necessary, tips and tricks to optimize the application are discussed. The endpoint of therapy is defined by the patient's individual decision, which is confirmed by our clinical examination during the routine outpatient clinic visit. In addition to the daily vacuum bell application, all our patients are recommended to carry on undertaking sports and physiotherapy, so that the accompanying improvement of body control results an important factor in outcome.

Patients

Our patients group comprises applicants aged from 3 to 61 years. As mentioned previously, we observed age specific differences of success [39], and therefore the most favourable age for this treatment has still to be defined.

During the first few applications, most of the patients experience moderate pain in the sternum. Adolescent and older patients develop moderate subcutaneous hematoma, which disappears within a few hours. Temporary side effects like transient paresthesia of the upper extremities during the application and/or mild dorsalgia are reported by some patients. These symptoms disappear when lower atmospheric pressure is used during application. Analgesic medication should not be necessary and has not been reported from any patient and parents, respectively. As mentioned above, the application of the vacuum bell in children aged 3–10 years should be supervised by parents or caregivers.

Results

Within the last 11 years, 300 patients (62 female, 238 male) started with vacuum bell treatment at our institution. The median age was 16.2 years (3–61 years). When starting with the application, 67/300 patients were above the age of 17 years, 58/300 above the age of 18 years. We published preliminary results of a subset of our patients group in 2011 [38]. Latest and more detailed results were summarized in another published study [39]. Hundred and forty patients (112 males, 28 females), aged 3–61 years (median 16.05 years) used the vacuum bell for 6 to maximum 69 months (average 20.5 months). When starting with the application, patients presented with a PE with depth from 1 to 6.3 cm (average 2.7 cm). After 3 months of treatment an elevation of more than 1 cm was documented in approx. 80 % of patients.

Daily application of the whole group was 107.9 min/day (range, 10–480 min). Application was terminated after 20.5 months. In 61 patients, the sternum was lifted to a normal level after 21.8 months (range, 6–69 months) (Figs. 17.4 and 17.5).

The follow-up after discontinuation is 27.6 months (range, 1–73 months), and the success until today is permanent and still visible (Figs. 17.4 and 17.5). Patients were very well motivated and compliant which is a basic precondition for a successful therapy. At follow-up, all patients were satisfied and expressed their motivation to continue the application, if necessary. Fifty-four patients are still under treatment. However, 25/140 patients stopped the application after 15.7 months (range, 1–42 months), due to an unsatisfactory result and/or decreasing motivation. 15/25 patients underwent MIRPE. The relevance of motivation was confirmed by the fact that 15 patients who underwent MIRPE, used the vacuum bell for 160.6 min/day whereas the remaining 10 patients who stopped any kind of therapy, used the vacuum bell for 36.3 min/day. In three patients with asymmetric PE, the depth of PE has decreased after 9 months, but the asymmetry is still visible (Fig. 17.6).

Intraoperative Use

Our experience with the vacuum bell method encouraged us to use the device intraoperatively during the MIRPE procedure to facilitate the dissection of the transmediastinal tunnel and the advancement of the pectus introducer, the riskiest step of the MIRPE procedure. As already demonstrated by Schier and Bahr for the first time [20], the elevation of the sternum is obvious and persists for a distinct period of time after application of the vacuum bell. Therefore, we considered that the vacuum cup may also be useful in reducing the risk of injury to the heart and the mammary vessels during the MIRPE procedure. Since the manufacturer of the device did not apply for the

approval to sterilize the vacuum bell until today, this additional use had to be considered as "Off-label". In agreement with our hospital hygienist and bearing in mind the nature of the material, we used gas sterilization for preparation of the device for intraoperative use.

Results

In a pilot study performed from 2005 to 2010, 50 patients aged from 9 to 28 years (average 14.95 years; 39 males and 11 females) were operated on for PE using the MIRPE procedure. Thirty-eight patients underwent primary surgery. Twelve patients (11 male, 1 female) used the vacuum bell for a period of 4–36 months (average 19.9 months) before surgery, and discontinued the

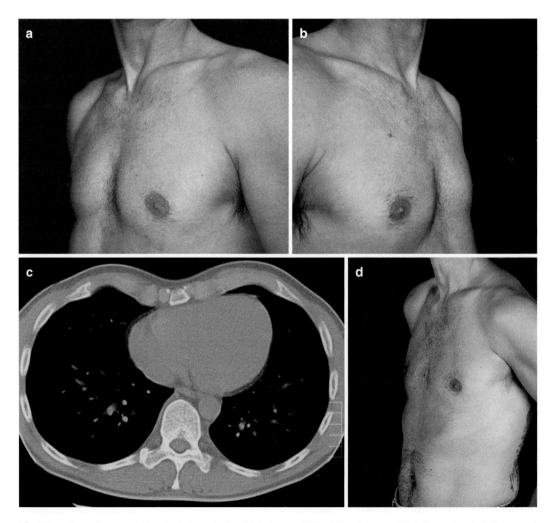

Fig. 17.4 Forty-five-year-old patient. (**a–c**) before (*left*: depth of PE = 2.5 cm) vacuum bell therapy and (**d–f**) after 12 months (*right*: depth of PE = 0.5 cm)

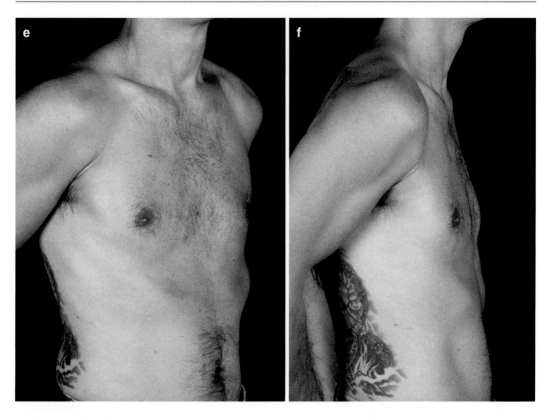

Fig. 17.4 (continued)

application due to decreasing motivation and/or insufficient success. The vacuum bell was applied for retrosternal dissection and advancement of the pectus introducer as well as placement and flipping of the pectus bar. The use of the vacuum bell led to a clear elevation of the sternum and this was confirmed by thoracoscopy (Fig. 17.7). Advancement of the pectus introducer and placement of the pectus bar was safe, successful and without adverse events in all patients. No evidence of cardiac and/or pericardiac lesions or lesions of the mammary vessels were noted intraoperatively by using right sided thoracoscopy. Additionally, no midline incision to elevate the sternum with a hook was necessary [22].

Discussion

A more differentiated analysis of our patients group will enable us "to see behind the curtain". Age and gender specific differences, depth of PE, symmetry or asymmetry, concomitant malformations like

scoliosis and/or kyphosis, etc. may influence the clinical course and the success of this therapy. The influence of individual motivation on the success has been described above.

However, there still remain some unanswered questions:

Optimal age for vacuum bell therapy The optimal age for this treatment has still to be defined. We observe age specific differences of success. In our experience, growth spurt during puberty is the most important period to influence degree and depth of PE. We started a pilot study using a measuring device which might enable us to measure the correlation between patients age, the depth of PE and the elevation of the chest wall during application. With these results, we may evaluate whether beginning with the vacuum therapy before puberty will be more useful than starting during puberty or even later.

Quantitative Measurement of Pressure The success of a therapeutic procedure not only requires a

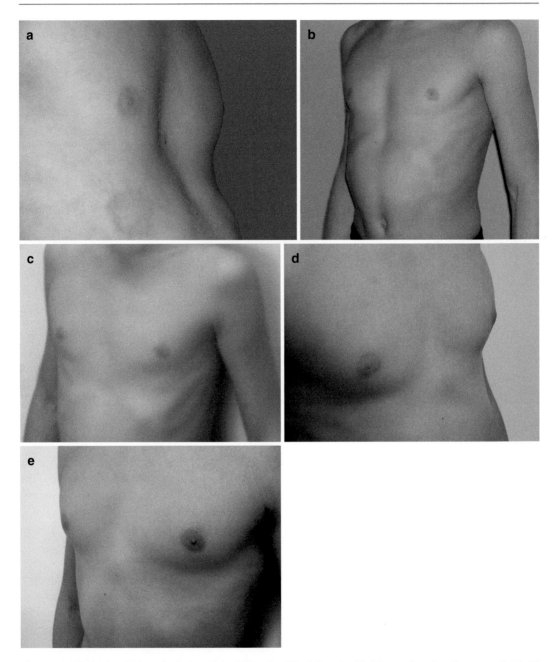

Fig. 17.5 Nine year old boy, (**a**) before (*left*: depth of PE = 2.8 cm) vacuum bell therapy, (**b**) after 10 months (*right*: depth of PE = 1.6 cm), (**c**) after 16 months (depth of PE: 0.4 cm), (**d**) 24 months after therapy and (**e**) 36 months after therapy

good technique, but also depends on an appropriate indication. It would be useful to measure the pressure that is necessary to lift the sternum during the first application. This measurement would enable us to divide patients into different groups, to identify suitable patients, and allow us to predict more accurately who of the users will benefit from this method and in whom the method will not work. As mentioned above, we are working on such a device to measure the pressure under the vacuum bell.

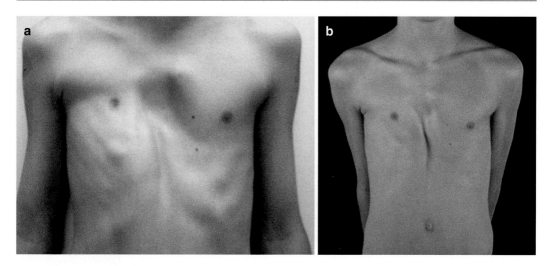

Fig. 17.6 Ten year old boy with asymmetric PE, before (**a**) vacuum bell therapy, and after 12 months (**b**)

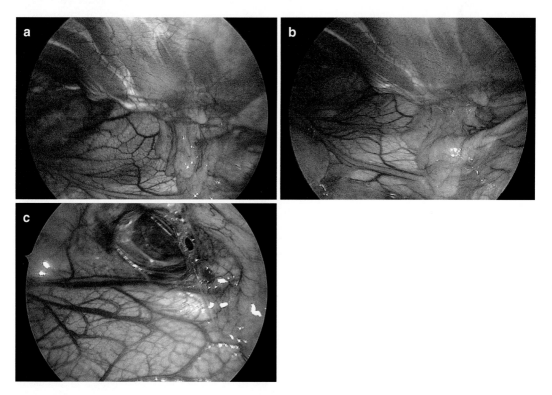

Fig. 17.7 Retrosternal space creation without (**a**) and with the vacuum bell (**b**) during the MIRPE procedure. (**c**) Note the retrosternal tunnel (**R**)

Supervision of daily application Until today, we have no possibility to supervise the frequency, the intensity and the duration of the daily application at home. Electronic devices which might be integrated into the vacuum bell, would be useful to supervise the routine application.

Long-term Results Long-term results including 10 years and more are still missing. Further studies are necessary to elucidate these facts.

Costs of Treatment In most European countries, costs of treatment have to be paid by patients and parents, respectively. In some countries in South America, acquisition of the vacuum bell is covered by the individual national health care system or the local insurance. In USA, approval of the FDA was obtained in May 2012.

Pre-Treatment before Surgery Physicians and patients discuss about the benefit to use the vacuum bell preoperatively prior to MIRPE procedure. Since in our country the majority of patients have to pay for the device, most of our patients are not interested in this "pre-treatment". Additionally, we observed no significant difference between patients who used the vacuum bell before surgery, and patients who underwent primary surgery [22].

Objective Assessment of Depth of PE To estimate the "objective" success of this treatment modality is very difficult. The definition of success may vary considerably between individuals. Depth of PE, symmetric vs. asymmetric deformity, as well as patients' age and sex represent important variables. Various scales and measurement methods including X-rays and computed tomography have been used to quantify the degree of deformity. Our method of assessment of depth of PE is not exact enough, especially regarding the age specific differences. New methods for non-invasive assessment of chest wall growth may provide more detailed, objective information concerning the severity of PE. A 3-D laser scanner might help us to assess the degree of PE and to follow-up our patients during vacuum therapy.

Pectus Carinatum

Introduction

PC is more frequent in males than females (4:1 ratio) and can be both symmetric or asymmetric. Rarely, the defect might be associated to Currarino-Silverman, combined pectus carinatum/excavatum, and Poland, Marfan or Von Recklinghausen syndromes, among other connective tissue disorders. Even though its etiology is unknown, PC may be genetically linked considering its frequent occurrence in families [40].

Apart from the external appearance which most commonly concerns patients and families, the majority of children present with relatively mild symptoms; the most frequently reported are tenderness, bone pain or mild exercise intolerance. Even though psychosocial issues secondary to body image need to be promptly addressed in all cases, since the defect tends to become more severe during pubertal growth spurts, and may even worsen throughout adult life, the physiological concerns must take precedence without exception.

Despite the early work of Jaubert de Beaujeu et al. and Bianchi et al. [41, 42], the pioneers in non-operative treatments for PC – open surgery has been the treatment of choice over the last decades [2, 43, 44]. Most of the existing surgical procedures consist of modifications of the Ravitch technique that employ resection of the deformed costal cartilages along with sternal osteotomy [45]. Even though patients refer to be generally pleased with the improvement of their chest's shape, surgery could not address the usual problem of the flaring of ribs and a visible scar was always left. On top of that, it is well known now, that surgery does not result in complete thorax remodeling in comparison to non-operative treatments. Many different authors proposed less radical resections [46–48].

Drs. Haje DP, Haje SA and coworkers from Brazil, have shared their valuable, extensive experience in treating PC patients using a Dynamic Compressor System (DCS) [49–52]. This was the consequence of four basic facts: (1) the inherent risks of a major surgery, (2) always reserved for the most severe cases, (3) leaving a great deal of patients untreated [53], in addition to (4) anterior chest wall compliance during puberty which permits remodeling by applying external compression. Based on the latter, other authors have also suggested a wide variety of alternative non-operative approaches [10–16], too.

The FMF® Dynamic Compressor System

Foreword

The Nuss procedure for pectus excavatum introduced a paradigm shift by demonstrating that the thoracic wall is a very elastic and malleable structure in children [9]. Inspired by this concept, early in the year 1999, the author and his partner, began assessing chest wall compliance in patients with mild to moderate forms of PC by applying manual compression to the defect. Since it could be corrected without pain, a non-operative prospective study was designed and implemented (after being approved by the institution's Research Ethics Committee) at the chest wall deformities outpatient clinic. A DCS was developed and utilized for this purpose. Besides, since by that time, there were no reports about the record and analysis of pressure measurements to compare series of patients, further investigation was done on that particular topic. By the beginning of 2001, the DCS design was finished. In 2008, the initial experience with the so-called FMF® Dynamic Compressor System (FMF stands for Fraire/Martinez-Ferro) was published [17–19]. Two quantifiable variables were defined to statistically compare objective data, collected at every consultation:

- **Pressure of Correction** (**POC**): the pressure applied to the patient until the proper shape of the thorax is achieved. Basically, it is an indirect parameter to measure and quantify the patient's chest wall flexibility. It is reduced throughout the treatment and is measured initially (because one of the inclusion criterions for bracing is that the POC ought to be equal or less than 14 PSI to prevent treatment failure) and at every consultation (Fig. 17.8).
- **Pressure of Treatment** (**POT**): the pressure required to treat the patient. It is measured before and after adjusting the FMF® DCS. POT permits evaluating whether the patient has been wearing the device or if he has grown up in between consultations. A POT higher than that obtained at the last consultation, means that he has not been wearing the brace as indicated, or that he has grown up (this can be verified by checking the registered height and weight or if the brace is too tight). Variables are recorded at an evolution form (Fig. 17.9).

First Projects

At first, different kinds of plastic and then metallic orthotic devices that proved to be inefficient were developed. It could be noticed that when the

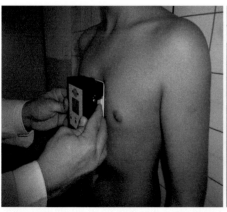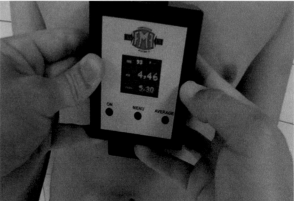

Fig. 17.8 Measurement of the **P**ressure **O**f **C**orrection (**POC**) at the first and successive consultations. The patient stands up against the wall. The pressure measuring device (PMD) is placed over the chest, where the protrusion is more prominent, and measures the pressure required to remodel the thorax. The initial POC helps to predict treatment duration and indirectly quantifies thoracic flexibility

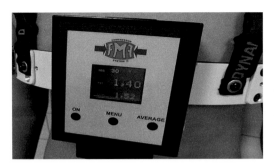

Fig. 17.9 Measurement of the **P**ressure **O**f **T**reatment (**POT**). Before and after adjustments to the FMF® DCS. Note the three buttons for optimum performance and the digital multiparameter color display of the **P**ressure **M**easuring **D**evice (**PMD**)

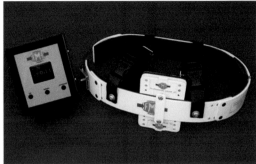

Fig. 17.10 Components of the FMF® Dynamic Compressor System: (*left*) **P**ressure **M**easuring **D**evice (**PMD**) and (*right*) aluminum, lightweight brace

patient's thorax was compressed, it expanded laterally. The team concluded the reason for their failure was the fact that thoracic lateral expansion, occurring naturally during inspiration, had not been taken into account.

With the aid of mechanical and electronic engineers, an external DCS was designed, but this time loaded with an electronic Pressure Measuring Device (PMD) to measure the POC and POT. The PMD converts the mechanical energy exerted to the patient (pressure) into electrical energy visible as numbers in a screen (measurement of pressure).

The unit of measurement to quantify pressure was decided to be pounds per square inch (PSI) because it takes into consideration the pressure resulting from a force of one pound-force applied to an area of one square inch. Presently, this is the unit of pressure that is still being employed. Most of the patients can be included with a decimal scale from 1 to 14.

By that time, the FMF® DCS included an expandable aluminum brace and the PMD.

The initial results obtained from measurements of POC, age, time of usage and cosmesis were analyzed from prospective collected data. Surprisingly, by correlating the different variables, the authors found out they could predict treatment duration and prognosis. These data has been very useful since then, to assess the patient and family about the treatment from the very first day of consultation.

Throughout the following years, several modifications were introduced to the FMF® DCS. The posterior compression pad was removed as it was not useful and caused skin lesions upon the spine and dorsal tissue. Better tolerance from PC patients could be enhanced to complete the treatment. A docking mechanism was designed to attach the PMD to the brace (for regulation of POT), in addition to a locking system, to avoid patient manipulation, and a portable plate bender to model the aluminum pieces.

Today

The FMF® DCS is currently a system comprised of the following elements:

1. A custom-fitted, expandable, low-profile (invisible under the patients' shirt), cushioned aluminum brace that is adjustable to any thoracic shape or size (Fig. 17.10). Its locking mechanism is situated on the side where the prominence is most evident to enhance compression. In order to avoid referrals, the brace has been designed to be ordered, assembled and implemented at different, distant locations with ease (Fig. 17.11). It permits lateral expansion to allow thorax widening as a consequence of breathing, growth and thoracic re-shaping (Fig. 17.12).
2. Different sizes and shapes of cushioned compression plates adaptable to distinctive sternal protrusions, independently of their locations, sizes and shapes (Fig. 17.13a);
3. Different compression pads that can be adhered to the compression plate to cushion

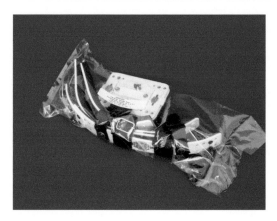

Fig. 17.11 Components of the FMF® Dynamic Compressor System: pieces to assemble a customized brace for each patient. Format in which they are delivered in a personalized packaging

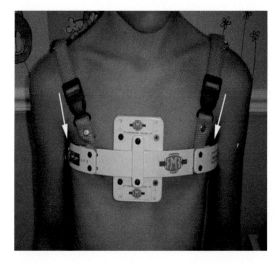

Fig. 17.12 The FMF® DCS enables lateral expansion during breathing and thoracic widening that occurs with re-shaping and growth. Note that at least a 1 cm space is left on each thoracic side. Basically the skin should not be in direct contact with the brace's undersurface to permit thoracic widening

the defect, prevent skin lesions, avoid non-compliance, increase POT in girls with breast development or when extra pressure needs to be exerted over the defect (Fig. 17.13b);

4. The PMD which can be docked to the brace's compression plate. Because of the variation of pressure when the PC patient inspires, the device latest version calculates the average POC and POT of multiple measurements taken in 5 s (Fig. 17.8).

5. Standardized measuring instruments (chest measuring ruler and metric tape) to record the data needed to assemble each brace (Fig. 17.14);

6. A portable plate bender to curve the aluminum segments according to the patient's continuous re-shaping thoracic anatomy (Fig. 17.15);

7. Specific tools as screwdrivers and screws (Fig. 17.14).

How Does it Work?

The FMF® DCS corrects PC by pushing the sternum backwards: the continuous anterior–posterior compression progressively widens and re-models the entire chest. Cartilages accommodate, grow and finally ossify in the correct position. The multiple aluminum segments can be adjusted, bent and eventually replaced at every consultation to permit proper lateral thoracic expansion, because an excessively tight brace causes non-compliance and treatment interruption.

The non-operative therapy consists of four distinct phases.

Initial Phase PC patients referred to the clinic are evaluated and those who meet the inclusion criteria (typical condrogladiolar pectus carinatum, POC < 14 PSI, consent to follow the treatment) are asked to join an institutional approved prospective study. A series of questions to reunite information for medical and academic purposes are made. Pictures are taken in six different positions (Fig. 17.16). Measurements to assemble the brace are filled in an order form.

Correction Phase Once the FMF® DCS is assembled and delivered to the patient, POT during maximal inspiration, and time of usage are set according to Table 17.1. POT over 2.5 PSI must be avoided since skin lesions can occur. The correction phase ends when the interdisciplinary team, patient, and/or family agree that the deformity has been fully repaired.

Originally PC patients were indicated to wear the brace as much as possible during the day (ideally 24 h per day). However, in order to enhance

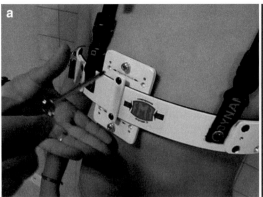
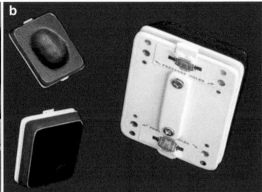

Fig. 17.13 Components of the FMF® Dynamic Compressor System (**a**) Adjustable compression plate. It is displaced frequently as the defect is compressed and its size, site and shape changes overtime. (**b**) Different sizes and shapes of cushioned compression pads designed for each type of protrusion to avoid skin lesions or to exert extra pressure (double or triple pads)

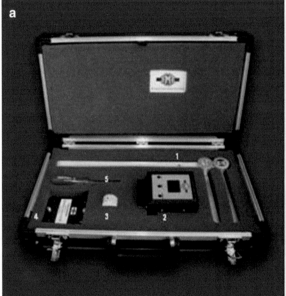
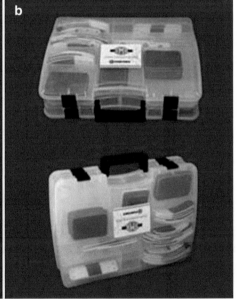

Fig. 17.14 Components of the FMF® Dynamic Compressor System. (**a**) Portable suitcase with standardized measuring instruments. Ref: (1) Measuring ruler; (2) PMD; (3) Measuring tape; (4) Removable compression plate; (5) Screwdrivers and screws. (**b**) Portable suitcases with the differently used and replacement pieces

compliance and to avoid skin lesions, PC patients have been currently classified into four distinct groups according to their initial POC. Once the patient's POC lowers to the POC range of the previous group, he is re-classified accordingly. Nonetheless, the treatment can be customized for each PC patient regarding tolerance, characteristic of the defect, skin status and age.

Following (Table 17.1) group 1 and 2 patients are instructed to wear the FMF® DCS every day, overnight and as much as possible during the day, depending on their activities. They are only allowed to remove the device during sports and while having a shower/bath. On the other hand, those PC patients belonging to group 3 and 4, commence wearing the system less hours per

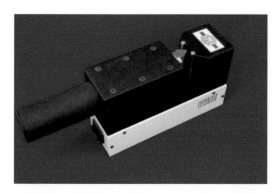

Fig. 17.15 Component of the FMF® Dynamic Compressor System. Portable plate bender to remodel aluminum lightweight pieces

day, at lower POTs, to indirectly increase the flexibility of the thoracic cage, to enhance compliance and to prevent skin lesions.

Group I and II PC patients are reminded at every consultation that the more they wear the FMF® DCS during the day and overnight, the faster their defect will be reverted.

Group III and IV are advised about the complications of overusing the brace and the need to follow medical indications.

A series of daily physical therapy exercises can be indicated, too. Swimming, playing wind instruments and inflating balloons (to treat the costal flares) are encouraged as accessory activities to complement the non-operative treatment.

A double-blinded patient-physician or family-physician survey has been implemented to assess final cosmetic results.

Basically, at the end of the correction phase, patients and/or parents (depending on age) are asked to judge the final outcome by assigning a score from 1 (poor) to 10 (excellent). Each treating physician of the interdisciplinary team submits an undisclosed judgment, too. The lowest 2 numbers are used to determine the final aesthetic result.

Printed (Fig. 17.16) and on-line historical pictures of each patient are always available at any time for consultation.

Weaning phase Once the defect is reverted, the FMF® DCS is gradually withdrawn to avoid eventual partial recurrences. PC may return mildly, in approximately 10 % of cured patients, particularly if they have been treated before pubertal growth spurts or in case they have cured very rapidly.

During the weaning phase, patients wear the brace as a "retainer" during the day or overnight (they generally prefer the latter), every day for the first month, every 2 days for the second month and every 3–4 days for the next months (range: 2–6 months). The weaning period is not contemplated in the calculation of the duration of treatment.

As aforementioned, the faster the patient gets cured, the longer the weaning phase should be. POT remains invariable in this post-correction period whilst POC is equal to cero.

Follow-up Phase Provisory treatment interruption is indicated when the weaning period ends. Patients are controlled every 6 months until they are 18 years old. In case of adults, treatment finishes when the defect is corrected. In any case, they are always indicated to call the office back if they observe any partial recurrence, that is, the appearance of a slight protrusion (never as prominent as the initial defect), which is corrected by adapting the brace to the new thoracic shape and a few more months of treatment.

Treatment Failure

Upon treatment failure or for those patients who are unlikely to be compliant with bracing, surgery is always an option (Fig. 17.17).

If the patient's chest is symmetrical and POC < 10 PSI, PC patients can be operated on with the Abramson technique which, consists of the insertion of subcutaneous and submuscular bars and stabilizers [47]. In most of the asymmetrical cases, even though an Abramson procedure can be tried, a classic thoracoplasty (using a modified Ravitch technique) is rather opted. The same is the case for those PC patients who additionally have a very stiff chest (POC > 10 PSI) or a failed previous surgery.

Results

Between April 2001 and October 2014, 500 patients were prescribed the staged, non-operative

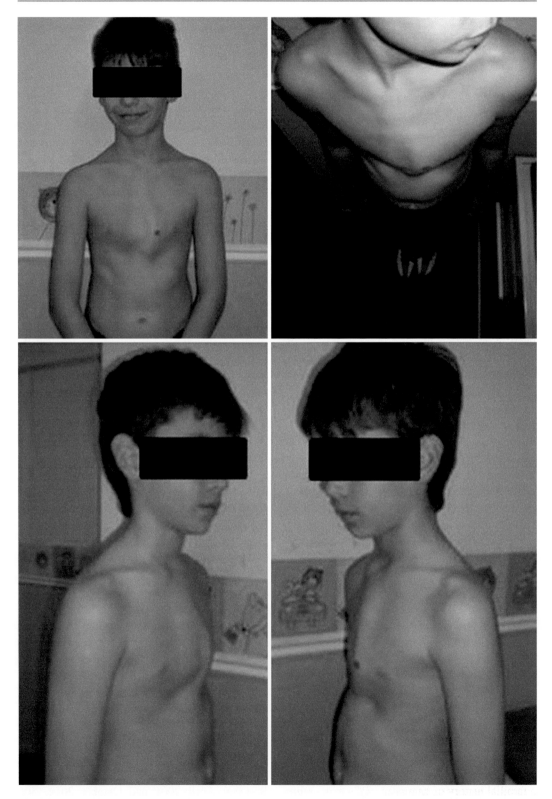

Fig. 17.16 Patient's medical record. Six pictures are taken at the first consultation (Front, From the top, 3/4 Right Side, 3/4 Left Side, Right Side, Left Side)

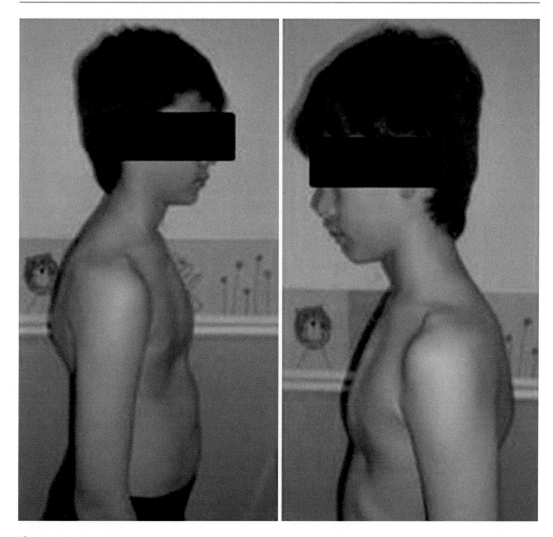

Fig. 17.16 (continued)

treatment, with the FMF® DCS and counseled to follow the protocol. Three hundred and eighty were males (76 %) and the mean age of detection of the defect was 12 ± 2 years (range: 1–34 years). Thirty-two patients (6.4 %) abandoned treatment and could not be evaluated for final results. Of these, 2 declared pain and 4 reported skin intolerance as the cause of noncompliance; the other 23 claimed social discomfort, and 3 patients were lost to follow-up. Of the remaining 468 patients, 398 completed the treatment (85 %), and 70 (15 %) are still actively using the FMF® DCS.

Seventy percent of patients (n = 328) reported a familial history of chest wall deformities. Fifty percent of patients were diagnosed scoliosis,

posterior asymmetry and a tendency to adopt a kyphotic position (n = 234). Forty percent of patients had asymmetric shoulders (n = 188) whereas 20 % of them evidenced costal flares (n = 94). Hundred percent of patients older than 8 years old referred social discomfort and feelings of embarrassment.

The mean time of use per patient (once adapted to treatment) was 18 ± 3 h per day for a mean period of 8 ± 5 months (range 3–24 months). When applying the satisfaction scale, 385 (97 %) patients achieved a 7- to 10-point correction (excellent, very good, and good results) and 13 (3 %), only 1- to 6 -point correction (poor and bad results). The mean initial POC value was 5 ± 1.5 PSI (range

Table 17.1 Treatment indicated at the first day of usage, until the patient tolerates the device without complications (pain, skin lesion, etc) or until the patient is re-classified into the previous group

Variables	Group 1	Group 2	Group 3	Group 4
Initial PC (PSI)	1–4	4–6	6–8	>8
Initial PT (PSI)	2.5	2	1.5	1
POT (PSI)	Reassigned according to the measured PC at every consultation until the patient tolerates full treatment			
Indicated time of usage (h)	24	24	12	6
Estimated treatment duration (months)	2	4	8	12–24

The treatment can vary among patients and be customized depending on compliance, site and height of the protrusion, sternal rotation, skin status and age

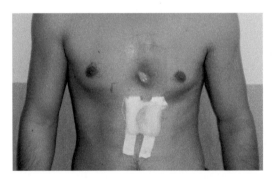

Fig. 17.17 Patient with skin ulceration caused by overusing the FMF® DCS beyond medical indication. The system was withdrawn until the lesion healed. The patient could soon employ the system as originally indicated and is currently in the weaning period

1–14 PSI). The following complications were observed in 20 of the 398 patients (5 %): back pain ($n=9$), hematoma ($n=1$), and skin lesions ($n=10$). No other complications were seen or reported. Even though complications caused a delay in completion of treatment, they were not the cause of treatment termination. Skin lesions were mild in all cases and treated by withdrawal of the FMF® DCS and/or topical skin lotions until the skin healed

completely. The other complications were treated by temporary loosening the FMF® DCS to lower the POT. Some patients with sensitive skin were indicated to wear a DuoDerm® Extra Thin patch at the site of the defect and/or a cotton shirt well adjusted to the body. There was a case of an adult patient who came to the clinic with a skin ulceration (Fig. 17.18). Skin ulcerations may happen in patients with extremely sensitive skin, excessive brace usage beyond medical indication -as was the case of the aformentioned patient- or in those patients with sharp protuberances (contoured compression pads were specifically designed to prevent skin lesions in the latter cases).

Follow-up ranged from 14 years to 1 month. During the follow-up, 40 patients (10 %) presented with a partial recurrence. These were mostly observed during periods of rapid growth and typically 6 ± 2 months after treatment discontinuance. All partial recurrences were mild, and successfully treated with the FMF® DCS, by modifying its shape and size to suit the patient's larger and widened thorax. All patients responded adequately and were promptly cured. Currently, in order to reduce partial recurrences, those patients who get corrected rapidly (less than 3 months), in particular, those with a low initial POC (Group I and II patients), are indicated a longer weaning period (up to 6 months).

Analysis of Results

The statistical studies adopted were the Independent samples Student's t-test for univariate analysis and the Regression analysis for multivariate analysis. Statistical significance was set at $p<0.01$. The statistical software program employed was SAS, version 8.02.

The collected pressure data denoted several interesting facts. POC is correlated with age ($p<0.01$), final cosmetic results ($p<0.01$), and treatment duration ($p<0.01$). Younger patients have a lower POC (major thoracic flexibility) than older patients. Better final cosmesis is observed in PC patients with a lower POC. The duration of treatment could be predicted at the time of the very first

Fig. 17.18 Treatment algorithm for pectus carinatum

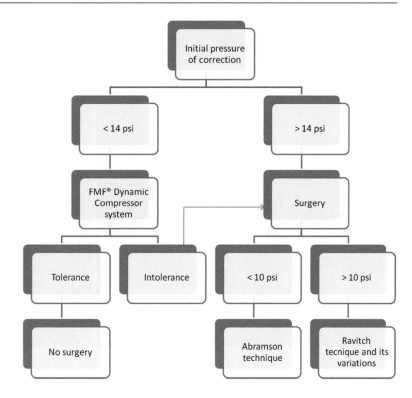

consultation. The duration of treatment is shorter in PC patients with more elastic and malleable thoraces (lower POCs) who wear the brace 24 h daily (except for showering, bathing and sports).

Regarding the pressure data, Group I patients can be cured in approximately 1–3 months (Fig. 17.19) whereas those belonging to Group II, get corrected in 3–4 months, and cured in 6 (Fig. 17.20). Group III patients are generally cured in 1 year (Fig. 17.21). Those in Group IV need between 15 and 24 months to revert their PC (Fig. 17.22). Upon treatment failure, the FMF® DCS softens the anterior chest and may facilitate surgery.

Correlation between POC and the duration of treatment results very useful in helping patients understand what is going to happen to them throughout the treatment.

Less than 2 % of PC patients (in particular Group I patients) show a tendency to overcorrection to PE. The treatment is immediately stopped in these cases, in whom the mild PE reverts spontaneously.

Chest X-ray, CT scan or a Chest MRI are not routinely indicated, unless the patient presents with an atypical PC, a stiff PC which demands further investigation, severe pain, or in case of an insecure family.

Throughout the correction phase, patients are monitored with a monthly frequency because of the need to adjust the brace, to verify the skin's status, to enhance the practice of complementary activities and brace wearing and to prevent overcorrection to PE.

Continuous Improvement Process

New projects are currently being developed to improve the FMF® DCS and to reduce data recollection bias. In a common project with the University of California, San Francisco, a time sensor, activated with body temperature, is being developed to measure the real "using time". An FMF® software is moreover being designed to process the measurable and applicable data, with implications for prognosis and treatment of PC [54].

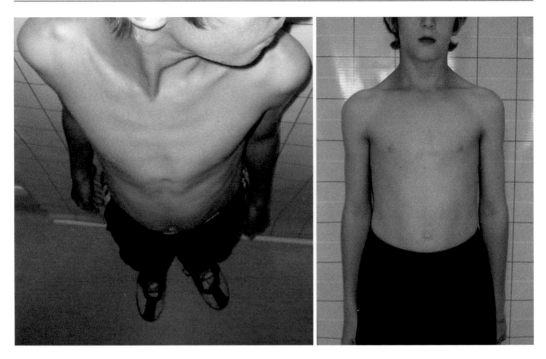

Fig. 17.19 Group 1 patient. Age: 9 years old. Initial PC = 3 PSI. 20 h of daily usage. Flat chest after 2 months

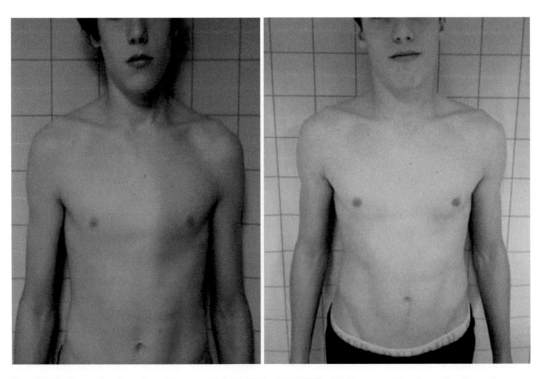

Fig. 17.20 Group 2 patient. Age: 14 years old. Initial PC = 5 PSI. 20 h of daily usage. Flat chest after 4 months

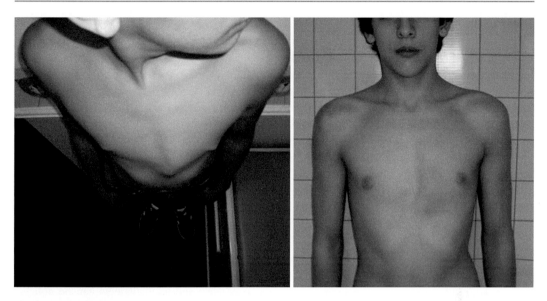

Fig. 17.21 Group 3 patient. Age 11 years old. Initial PC = 7 PSI. 15 h of daily usage. Flat chest after 8 months

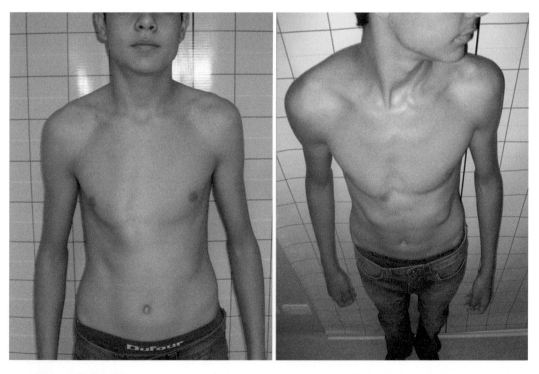

Fig. 17.22 Group 4 patient. Age: 16 years old. Initial PC = 9 PSI. 18 h of daily usage. Flat chest after 1 year. Note that the higher the age and initial PC, in addition to the presence of sternal rotation, the less optimum is the cosmetic result. Anyway the patient reported a satisfaction score of 9

Discussion

The non-operative treatment for PC essentially mirrors the effects of the internal bar in PE patients, remodeling the growth pattern of the deformed chest wall cartilages [16, 55]. By the year 1999, except for the pioneer papers of Haje et al. [49–52] no other authors supported a non-operative approach for the treatment of mild to moderate cases of PC [45, 53]. Simultaneously with Dr. Haje et al, but by that time unaware of their work, the author and his partner, began developing a DCS to treat PC conservatively. As aforementioned, the DCS design was finished in 2001.

Moreover, starting almost simultaneously with the author and colleagues, several other authors have suggested a diverse variety of non-operative approaches based on the same concept: that the anterior chest wall is still compliant during puberty and permits remodeling by applying external compression [11–15], reaching to similar results and conclusions. What differentiated the FMF® DCS from other devices was essentially that the POC and POT could be objectively measured using the PMD, enabling prediction of treatment duration and prognosis.

Our initial results have been validated by other surgeons as Dr. Cohee AS and her teamwork, who are treating patients amenable to bracing with the FMF® DCS, at the Children's Hospital of the King's Daughter in Norfolk, USA [56]. They have reported very good results and observed that one of the system's advantage over other orthotics, is that it objectively measures the POC and POT to guide treatment decisions. Because the position of the compression plate is early adjusted on the aluminum frame, flattening of the sternum is enhanced in asymmetric cases is enhanced. Many other authors have recently validated our initial results [57–60].

When comparing historical open surgery results with those of the non-operative treatment, the benefits of the latter are superlative. To begin with, the FMF® DCS not only remodels the sternum and cartilaginous ribs permanently, but also results in complete thoracic re-shaping in contrast to an operation. Secondly, it totally eliminates the risks of anesthesia and of major surgeries, decreasing the complication rate, leaving no visible scar, avoiding hospital admission, avoiding activity restrictions associated to implant placing and dramatically reducing the cost of treatment. When considering the benefits of a non-operative treatment, almost no patient with a POC equal or less than 14 PSI should be selected as a candidate for surgery before trying a conservative approach.

Conclusion

The vacuum bell therapy may help to avoid surgery in some patients with PE. Specially younger patients with symmetric and mild PE may benefit from this procedure. The application is easy, and a good acceptance by both paediatric and adult patients can be noticed. However, a more differentiated analysis must focus on age and gender specific differences to help identify appropriate patients. Moreover, the time of follow-up with a maximum of 10 years is still not long enough, and further follow-up studies are necessary to evaluate the effectiveness of this therapeutic tool.

The intraoperative use of the vacuum bell during the MIRPE facilitates the retrosternal dissection and advancement of the pectus introducer as well as placement and flipping of the pectus bar. It leads to a clear elevation of the sternum without adverse events in all patients, as cardiac and/or pericardiac lesions or lesions of the mammary vessels. No midline incision to elevate the sternum with a hook is necessary. In any case, the method seems to be a valuable adjunct therapy in the treatment of PE.

The FMF® DCS permits thoracic lateral expansion (re-shaping), pressure measurement and control, prediction of treatment duration and prognosis, in-situ outpatient clinic adjustments, avoids patient manipulation and spine and dorsal injury, thereby providing increased tolerance. It can be indicated, placed and controlled by any physician at distant locations, who can additionally collect objective data to enable him adjust the FMF® DCS and perform further scientific evaluations. The implementation of a staged treatment, consisting of four distinctive phases allows patients to be treated non-operatively with optimum reversion of their PC and complete thoracic remodeling. Upon failure, open or video-surgery are always a viable alternative. As is the case of vacuum bells further follow-up studies are needed to evaluate the effectiveness of this therapeutic tool.

References

1. Ravitch MM. The operative treatment of pectus excavatum. Ann Surg. 1949;129(4):429–44.
2. Ravitch MM. The operative correction of pectus carinatum. Bull Soc Int Chir. 1975;34(2):117–20.
3. Robicsek F, Watts LT, Fokin AA. Surgical repair of pectus excavatum and carinatum. Semin Thorac Cardiovasc Surg. 2009;21(1):64–75.
4. Saxena AK, Willital GH. Valuable lessons from two decades of pectus repair with the Willital-Hegemann procedure. J Thorac Cardiovasc Surg. 2007;134(4):871–6.
5. Wang LS, Kuo KT, Wang HW, Yang CH, Chin T. A novel surgical correction through a small transverse incision for pectus excavatum. Ann Thorac Surg. 2005;80(5):1951–4.
6. Fonkalsrud EW. 912 open pectus excavatum repairs: changing trends, lessons learned: one surgeon's experience. World J Surg. 2009;33(2):180–90.
7. Kelly RE, Goretsky MJ, Obermeyer R, Kuhn MA, Redlinger R, Haney TS, Moskowitz A, Nuss D. Twenty-one years of experience with minimally invasive repair of pectus excavatum by the Nuss procedure in 1215 patients. Ann Surg. 2010;252(6):1072–81.
8. Pectus UP Surgery Kit. http://venturamedicaltechnologies.com/es/productos/pectus-up. Website visited on 1 Jan 2015.
9. Nuss D, Kelly Jr RE, Croitoru DP, et al. A 10-year review of a minimally invasive technique for the correction of pectus excavatum. J Pediatr Surg. 1998;33(4):545–52.
10. Kravarusic D, Dicken BJ, Dewar R, et al. The Calgary protocol for bracing of pectus carinatum: a preliminary report. J Pediatr Surg. 2006;41:923–6.
11. Banever GT, Konefal SH, Gettens K, et al. Nonoperative correction of pectus carinatum with orthotic bracing. J Laparoendosc Adv Surg Tech A. 2006;16:164–7.
12. Frey AS, Garcia VF, Brown RL, et al. Nonoperative management of pectus carinatum. J Pediatr Surg. 2006;41:40–5; discussion 40–5.
13. Egan JC, DuBois JJ, Morphy M, et al. Compressive orthotics in the treatment of asymmetric pectus carinatum: a preliminary report with an objective radiographic marker. J Pediatr Surg. 2000;35:1183–6.
14. Mielke CH, Winter RB. Pectus carinatum successfully treated with bracing. A case report. Int Orthop. 1993;17(6):350–2.
15. Stephenson JT, Du Bois J. Compressive orthotic bracing in the treatment of pectus carinatum: the use of radiographic markers to predict success. J Pediatr Surg. 2008;43(10):1776–80.
16. Lee SY, Lee SJ, Jeon CW, Lee CS, Lee KR. Effect of the compressive brace in pectus carinatum. Eur J Cardiothorac Surg. 2008;34(1):146–9.
17. Martinez-Ferro M, Fraire C, Bernard S. Dynamic compression system for the correction of pectus carinatum. Semin Pediatr Surg. 2008;17(3):194–200.
18. Martinez-Ferro M. International innovations in pediatric minimally invasive surgery: the Argentine experience. J Pediatr Surg. 2012;47(5):825–35.
19. Martinez-Ferro M. New approaches to pectus and other minimally invasive surgery in Argentina. J Pediatr Surg. 2010;45(1):19–26; discussion 26–7.
20. Schier F, Bahr M, Klobe E. The vacuum chest wall lifter: an innovative, nonsurgical addition to the management of pectus excavatum. J Pediatr Surg. 2005;40(3):496–500.
21. Haecker FM, Mayr J. The vacuum bell for treatment of pectus excavatum: an alternative to surgical correction? Eur J Cardiothorac Surg. 2006;29(4):557–61. Epub 2006 Feb 13.
22. Haecker FM, Sesia SB. Intraoperative use of the vacuum bell for elevating the sternum during the Nuss procedure. J Laparoendosc Adv Surg Tech A. 2012;22:934–6.
23. Nuss D, Croitoru DP, Kelly RE, Goretsky MJ, Nuss KJ, Gustin TS. Review and discussion of the complications of minimally invasive pectus excavatum repair. Eur J Pediatr Surg. 2002;12:230–4.
24. Haecker F-M, Bielek J, von Schweinitz D. Minimally invasive repair of pectus excavatum (MIRPE): the Basel experience. Swiss Surg. 2003;9:289–95.
25. Park HJ, Lee SY, Lee CS. Complications associated with the Nuss procedure: analysis of risk factors and suggested measures for prevention of complications. J Pediatr Surg. 2004;39:391–5.
26. Hosie S, Sitkiewicz T, Petersen C, Göbel P, Schaarschmidt K, Till H, et al. Minimally invasive repair of pectus excavatum – the Nuss procedure. A European multicentre experience. Eur J Pediatr Surg. 2002;12:235–8.
27. Berberich T, Haecker F-M, Kehrer B, Erb T, Günthard J, Hammer J, Jenny P. Postcardiotomy syndrome after minimally invasive repair of pectus excavatum. J Pediatr Surg. 2004;39:e1–3.
28. Van Renterghem KM, von Bismarck S, Bax NMA, Fleer A, Hoellwarth M. Should an infected Nuss bar be removed? J Pediatr Surg. 2005;40:670–3.
29. Barakat MJ, Morgan JA. Haemopericardium causing cardiac tamponade: a late complication of pectus excavatum repair. Heart. 2004;90:e22–3.
30. Barsness K, Bruny J, Janik JS, Partrick DA. Delayed near-fatal hemorrhage after Nuss bar displacement. J Pediatr Surg. 2005;40:E5–6.
31. Hoel TN, Rein KA, Svennevig JL. A life-threatening complication of the Nuss-procedure for pectus excavatum. Ann Thorac Surg. 2006;81:370–2.
32. Adam LA, Lawrence JL, Meehan JJ. Erosion of the Nuss bar into the internal mammary artery 4 months

after minimally invasive repair of pectus excavatum. J Pediatr Surg. 2008;43:394–7.

33. Gips H, Zaitsev K, Hiss J. Cardiac perforation by a pectus bar after surgical correction of pectus excavatum: case report and review of the literature. Pediatr Surg Int. 2008;24:617–20.

34. Haecker F-M, Berberich T, Mayr J, Gambazzi F. Near-fatal bleeding after transmyocardial ventricle lesion during removal of the pectus bar after the Nuss procedure. J Thorac Cardiovasc Surg. 2009;138(5): 1240–1. Epub 2008 Sep 19.

35. Lange F. Thoraxdeformitäten. In: Pfaundler M, Schlossmann A, editors. Handbuch der Kinderheilkunde, Vol V. Chirurgie und Orthopädie im Kindesalter. Leipzig: FCW Vogel; 1910. p. 157.

36. Spitzy H. Deformitäten der Wirbelsäule. In: Lange F, editor. Lerbuch der Orthopädie. Jena: Gustav Fischer; 1922.

37. Bahr M. Vacuum bell procedure according to Eckart Klobe (nonsurgical). In: Schwabegger A, editor. Congenital thoracic wall deformities. Springer. 1st ed. 2011.

38. Haecker F-M. The vacuum bell for conservative treatment of pectus excavatum. The Basle experience. Pediatr Surg Int. 2011;27:623–7.

39. Haecker F-M, Zuppinger J, Sesia S. Die konservative Therapie der Trichterbrust mittels Vakuumtherapie. Schweiz Med Forum 14 2014;(45):842–9.

40. Mégarbané A, Daou L, Mégarbané H, et al. New autosomal recessive syndrome with short stature and facio-auriculo-thoracic malformations. Am J Med Genet A. 2004;128:414–7.

41. Jaubert de Beaujeu M, et al. Thorax en carène. Lyon Chir. 1964;60:440–3.

42. Bianchi C, et al. Risultati a distanza 20 casi di "Cifosi Sternale" tratti incruentemente. Fracastoro. 1968;61: 779–92.

43. Welch KJ, Vos A. Surgical correction of pectus carinatum (pigeon breast). J Pediatr Surg. 1973;8:659–67.

44. Haller Jr JA. History of the operative management of pectus deformities. Chest Surg Clin N Am. 2000;10(2): 227–35.

45. Fonkalsrud EW, Beanes S. Surgical management of pectus carinatum: 30 years' experience. World J Surg. 2001;25:898–903.

46. Fonkalsrud EW, Anselmo DM. Less extensive techniques for repair of pectus carinatum: the undertreated chest deformity. J Am Coll Surg. 2004;198:898–905.

47. Abramson H. A minimally invasive technique to repair pectus carinatum. Preliminary report. Arch Bronconeumol. 2005;41:349–51.

48. Schaarschmidt K, Kolberg-Schwerdt A, Lempe M, et al. New endoscopic minimal access pectus carinatum repair using subpectoral carbon dioxide. Ann Thorac Surg. 2006;81:1099–103.

49. Haje SA, Bowen JR, Harcke HT, Guttenberg ME, et al. Disorders in the sternum growth and pectus deformities: an experimental model and clinical correlation. Acta Orthop Bras. 1998;6:67–75.

50. Haje SA, Bowen JR. Preliminary results of orthotic treatment of pectus deformities in children and adolescents. J Pediatr Orthop. 1992;12(6):795–800.

51. Haje SA, Harcke HT, Bowen JR. Growth disturbance of the sternum and pectus deformities: imaging studies and clinical correlation. Pediatr Radiol. 1999;29:334–41.

52. Haje A, Haje DP, Silva Neto M, et al. Pectus deformities: tomographic analysis and clinical correlation. Skeletal Radiol. 2010;39(8):773–82.

53. Fonkalsrud EW. Pectus carinatum: the undertreated chest malformation. Asian J Surg. 2003;26:189–92.

54. Harrison B, Stern L, Chung P, Etemadi M, Kwiat D, Harrison M, Martinez-Ferro M. MYPECTUS: a novel mobile health system for remote assessment of treatment. Presented at the American Pediatric Surgical Association annual meeting on 31 May, 2014 in Phoenix.

55. Lee RT, Moorman S, Schneider M, et al. Bracing is an effective therapy for pectus carinatum: interim results. J Pediatr Surg. 2013;48(1):184–90.

56. Cohee AS, Lin JR, Frantz FW, Kelly Jr RE. Staged management of pectus carinatum. J Pediatr Surg. 2013;48(2):315–20.

57. Lopez M, Patoir A, Varlet F, Perez-Etchepare E, Tiffet T, Villard A, Tiffet O. Preliminary study of efficacy of dynamic compression system in the correction of typical pectus carinatum. Eur J Cardiothorac Surg. 2013;44(5):e316–9.

58. Obermeyer RJ, Goretsky MJ. Chest wall deformities in pediatric surgery. Surg Clin North Am. 2012; 92(3):669–84.

59. Sesia S, Haecker F-M. Dynamisches Kompressionssystem bei Kielbrust - eine neuartige konservative Behandlungsmethode für Kinder und Jugendliche. Hausarzt Praxis. 2014;9(2):26–9.

60. de Beer SA, de Jong JR, Heij HA. Dynamische-compressiebrace bij pectus carinatum. Ned Tijdschr Geneeskd. 2013;157:159.

Patient Experience Before and After Treatment: Psychological Effects and Patients' Personal Experience

18

Shyam K. Kolvekar, Natalie L. Simon, and Trupti Kolvekar

Abstract

Pectus excavatum is the most frequent congenital anterior chest wall and sternal deformity. The NUSS procedure is a minimally-invasive surgical intervention carried out on patients with the anomaly. The procedure has an extremely high success rate and is proven to benefit the patient's respiratory and cardiac function. Pectus excavatum patients suffer frequent embarrassment over physical appearance and teasing- 22.8 % patients reported such teasing, with an expected 97.4 % majority of teasing coming from peers. Two patients were chosen, at either end of the age spectrum, and they shared an account of their own experiences.

Keywords

Chest wall deformity • Pectus Excavatum • Psychosocial Impact • Nuss Procedure • Pain Management

Pectus excavatum is the most frequent congenital anterior chest wall and sternal deformity. The NUSS procedure is the minimally invasive surgi-

S.K. Kolvekar, MS, MCh, FRCS, FRCSCTh (✉)
Department of Cardiothoracic Surgery,
University College London Hospitals, The Heart Hospital and Barts Heart Center, London, UK
e-mail: kolvekar@yahoo.com

N.L. Simon, MBBS
Department of School of Medical Education,
Kings College London, London, UK

T. Kolvekar, BSc Biochemistry (Hon)
The Department of Structural Molecular Biology,
University College London, London, UK

cal intervention carried out on patients with the anomaly. The procedure has an extremely high success rate and is proven to benefit the patient's respiratory and cardiac function. Another less-documented benefit observed post-surgery is the considerable improvement in psychological welfare and social interaction. The negative psychological impact of pectus excavatum on patients has been proven to cause sufficient distress and induce constant self-scrutiny. Research undertaken on patients measuring psychosocial status prior-to and after treatment warrants the need for surgery. Non-surgical treatment methods are also proven to be effective at improving the patient's emotional condition and physical satisfaction.

The majority of studies agree on the extent of poor psychological status amongst pectus excavatum patients. Eighty percent of patients observed in an n = 10 cohort study suffered psychological limitations, concerning *attractiveness, self-esteem and somatisation*. Eighty percent of the cohort was found to shy away from body presentation, for instance, when swimming or doing sports. The study found this to lead to insecurity, anxiety and denegation of the own body. Forty percent reported breathlessness, however, their lung-function tests were normal and there was no affirmed pulmonary limitation [1]. 74.8 % of patients in another study conducted to assess psychosocial functioning and its risk factors in children with pectus excavatum were found to have first perceived their deformity between 4 and 6 years of age. 58.8 % of patients in the study found the deformation by themselves and, comparatively less, (41.2 %) were informed of their deformation by people around them [2].

Pectus excavatum patients suffer frequent embarrassment over physical appearance and teasing- 22.8 % patients reported such teasing, with the expected 97.4 % majority of teasing coming from peers. This signals for information regarding pectus excavatum and other such chest deformities being implemented into the curriculum at educational establishments. Being teased about their chest deformity has proven to powerfully motivate patients to seek-out help regarding surgical and non-surgical treatment available. 37.1 % of patients actively sought help by asking their parents to take them to hospital [2]. Intermittent assiduity of the patient's physical appearance is said to cause a substantial lowering of one's self-esteem and extensive feelings of inferiority, depression, shyness and social anxiety. Poor body language is also discerned, such as a sloping posture with folded arms. Lifestyle restrictions often involve avoiding chest exposure when swimming, playing other sports, hugging and intimate relationships. In fact, 43.6 % of patients in the same cohort study admitted to finding chest exposure difficult and restraining from participation in such activities [2]. During puberty, the psychological strain due to pectus excavatum proved disadvantageous to development [1].

United Kingdom has a unique situation due to the National Health Service (NHS), which caters for the masses and is incredibly efficient at dealing with life-saving conditions. Often, in the past, when concerned parents approached their family General Practitioners with either funnel or pigeon chests, they were only reassured and not referred for any treatment. Some of these patients suffered in silence and it affected them in social environments. However, eventually patients started looking for answers; due to increased awareness of the condition, availability of treatment and the internet, leading to a large numbers of patients coming forward for first time to seek treatment. Treatment is available for early teens, depending on which region of the country the patient is from. There are a variety of reasons to why a patient would seek treatment from cosmetic, backaches to breathing issues, thus we see patients with either an unperturbed manner to extremely apprehensive and anxious attitude to their treatment (Table 18.1).

Patient Experience

AB: Male, 17 Years of Age

My experience of pectus excavatum and how I felt afterwards.

The main reason why I had the nuss technique surgery was cosmetic, although I was concerned that the condition might affect my lung capacity in the future even though I do not have respiratory problems now.

I first noticed when I was 13 years old in September 2011, my friends at school commented on it and I didn't really like that. We went away to Egypt that Christmas and my older brother pointed it out to me and I realised that it was quite severe. During the next 6 months it seemed to get worse. In summer 2012, I went to the doctor. I had looked it up by then and knew that I probably had a condition called 'pectus excavatum'. My GP said it was quite common but when I showed him my chest he did say that this was the worst case he had ever seen, and referred me to the hospital.

Table 18.1 Prevalence of psychosocial problems in patient group and control group

CBCL Scale	Patient group	Control group	x^2	P
	N = 337	N = 370		
Withdrawn	23 (6.82)	12 (3.24)	4.808	0.028[a]
Somatic complaints	15 (4.45)	8 (2.16)	2.692	0.087
Anxious/depressed	27 (8.01)	15 (4.05)	4.944	0.026[a]
Social problems	21 (6.23)	9 (2.43)	6.264	0.012[a]
Thought problems	17 (5.04)	12 (3.24)	1.455	0.228
Attention problems	16 (4.75)	13 (3.51)	0.683	0.409
Delinquent behavior	19 (5.64)	11 (2.97)	3.038	0.079
Aggressive behavior	21 (6.23)	13 (3.51)	2.846	0.092
Total problem	66 (19.58)	47 (12.70)	6.220	0.013[a]

From Ji et al. [2]. © 2011 Ji et al; licensee BioMed Central Ltd. This is an Open Access article distributed under the terms of the Creative Commons Attribution License (http://creativecommons.org/licenses/by/2.0), which permits unrestricted use, distribution, and reproduction in any medium, provided the original work is properly cited
Data are presented as number (%); CBCL: child behaviour checklist
[a]The differences are statistically significant if $P < 0.05$

That made me feel quite self conscious. Throughout the following year I was seen by a consultant a couple of time and had various photographs and tests. When I went on family holidays I did not like taking my t-shirt off which stopped me participating in some activities, for example swimming, that I would have done if it wasn't for my chest (Figs. 18.1, 18.2, and 18.3).

About a year after I had been diagnosed in summer 2013, I was expecting to have my operation, however my local hospital in Brighton does not do chest wall surgery on children so I had to wait for a place in London. My GSCE's intervened so I had to wait another year for my actual surgery.

The surgery went well although afterwards I was in a lot of pain, which is expected with this operation. I was on a morphine drip for a few days. The morphine made me very sick and also gave me hallucinations, which are common side effects. After I came off the morphine, I went onto oral pain relief. I recovered quite quickly after this and 3–4 weeks after surgery I was more or less off all pain relief. By this time I was also able to undertake light exercise, for example table tennis, going to the gym and riding my bike. About 2 months after surgery I started playing tennis, which is my favourite sport. For several weeks after the operation I was quite tired but within 5 or 6 weeks this stopped and I was able to carry on my normal routine (Figs. 18.4, 18.5, 18.6, and 18.7)

Overall I am very happy with the way my chest looks now, especially as I only had the operation a few months ago and I would recommend the operation to anyone. If I were in the same situation, I would definitely go through the process again. I feel much more confidant about taking my t-shirt off now, in fact I really like the way my chest looks now. There are still a couple of scars but these are already barely noticeable and I am not self-conscious about these at all.

I am planning a ski trip in February 2015.

AE: 48 Years of Age

I first became self-conscious about my pectus excavatum in my mid-teens. Prior to then, I had of course noticed that the shape of my rib-cage was different to that of most others, but had put this down to the fact that I was very skinny, and so the contours of my ribs were easier to see than most. My mother had often commented that my chest was just like that of her own father, my granddad.

Once I had realized that my ribcage was not "normal", life was never the same again.

Having never previously worried about clothes, I would now only wear loose-fitting tops, in dark colours, to better hide the dent and flared ribs. Swimming was a military-precise exercise, in which I would strive to get changed into trunks,

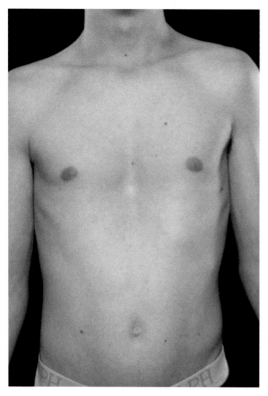

Fig. 18.1 Before: Front view

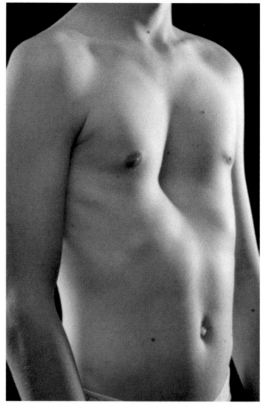

Fig. 18.2 Before: Right side view

and walk to the pool (arms crossed over my chest) without anyone seeing my chest, relaxing only once in the water. Girlfriends' hands were gently pushed away from by chest "because that tickles"; they would never see my naked chest, but instead plenty of dark coloured vests which became my trademark. At University, I remember buying two rolls of bandages in Freshers' Week, and trying to mummify my torso to improve its shape (it didn't work).

So, I was acutely aware and embarrassed by my chest's appearance. Of equal concern were the pains that would intermittently run down the inside of my left arm. I didn't know for sure, and still don't know, whether these were symptoms of my PE, but I assumed so, and this exacerbated my unhappiness and pre-occupation with the condition.

Over the years, it is true to say that my self-consciousness about my PE was never very far from the front of my mind. Before a social event, I would fret over the outfit that would least reveal

my chest-shape. Going out in a tee shirt on a windy day was a no-no – the wind would blow the shirt to the contours of my chest. Sea- or pool-side holidays with friends were out of the question – it would be just too difficult to keep my "secret" hidden.

One might think that as someone with PE gets older, that the self-consciousness lessens, that he or she gets a sense of perspective – "worse things happen at sea". This was not my experience. I remained as acutely concerned about it in my 20s, 30s and 40s as I was in my mid-to-late teens. The routines which I put in place to hide the PE, particular clothes types, arms crossed where circumstances demanded it, remained in place.

Before marrying my wife, I had relationships with several other women, none of who were ever aware that I had PE (I'm still not quite sure how I managed to achieve this).

I first met my wife when she and I were both 18, although we didn't marry until we were 31 (and had spent most of the years in between apart, and with other partners). She was the one (non-family) person in whom I was able to confide, although I still was not able to relax without a top on even in her company. It never bothered her at

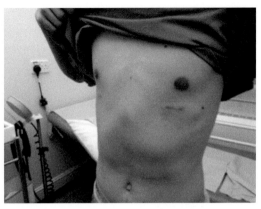

Fig. 18.5 After: left side view

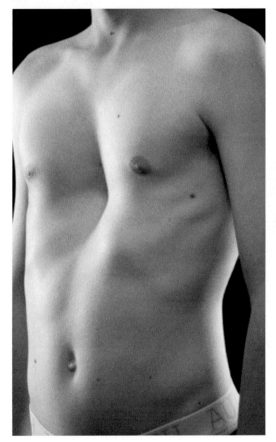

Fig. 18.3 After: Left side view

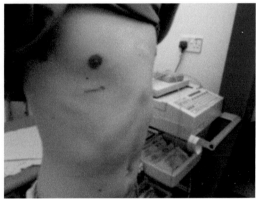

Fig. 18.6 After right side view

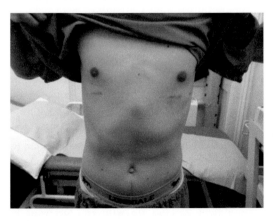

Fig. 18.4 After: Front view

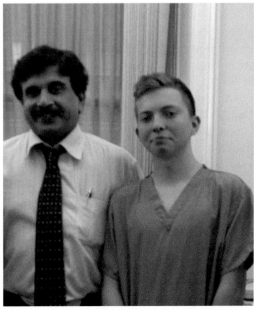

Fig. 18.7 The author and surgeon during work experience

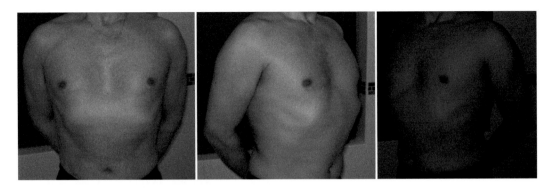

Fig. 18.8 Before surgery for pectus excavatum

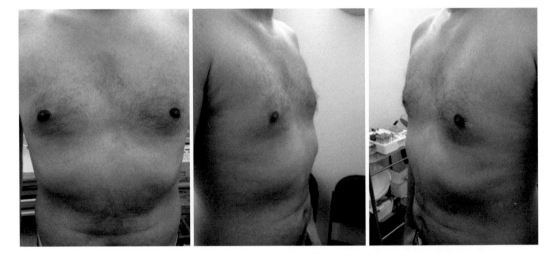

Fig. 18.9 After surgery for pectus excavatum

all; and she was always trying to reassure me that no-one would notice, which, whilst I appreciated the sentiment, didn't do anything to put my mind at rest.

Our first child, Daniel, was born on Valentine's Day 2000, our pride and joy. Within days I noticed a small hollow in his chest; I was distraught to see that I had passed on my condition to my first-born. We have since had a second son and a daughter, neither of who has PE; and, strangely enough, neither my younger sister nor my brother has PE.

I was 33 when Daniel was born, and had never considered that there might be a remedy for my condition. Indeed, at that time, I did not know that there was a medical name for the condition, that it was a condition shared by 1000s of others, and that indeed, there had been surgical proce-

dures to address the condition for many years. It was Daniel having PE that eventually prompted me, in around 2007, to research the condition as much as possible, and I quickly found the wonderful website www.pectusinfo.com and the wealth of information available on its forums.

In 2010, I became aware that Dr. Hans Pilegaard, a world-renowned surgeon specializing in the correction of pectus deformities, was making regular visits to the London Heart Hospital to work with Dr. Shyam Kolvekar on UK cases. I started to fantasize about a solution to my own condition, without ever really believing it would happen. And then I send an email to Dr Kolvekar, who replied within minutes suggesting I contact his (wonderful) PA, Amy Gooding. Email exchanges with Amy, and an appointment was set up with Dr. Kolvekar in

London, within weeks. During my appointment with Dr. Kolvekar, he was warm, friendly, and immediately sympathetic to my condition. A subsequent appointment was scheduled for tests to gauge my suitability for the Nuss operation. A brief wait for a date when Dr. Pilegaard would next be at the London Heart Hospital, and then, so soon after my first email to Dr Kolvekar, a letter with the date of my operation.

I was ecstatic.

The staff at London Heart Hospital is fantastic, and my memories of my 3-day stay there for the Nuss operation are of being extremely well looked after. I remember Dr. Kolvekar and Dr. Pilegaard coming to see me the night before the operation, debating briefly whether it was a one- or two-bar fix, and putting my mind to rest on the natural concerns I had. I just knew I was in the best hands.

Post-operation, once I was back on the ward, I barely dared to take a look at my chest. For 45 years when I'd looked down at my chest, my heart sank (literally and metaphorically!) and it was very hard to believe I was dent-free. The result surpassed my wildest expectations – my chest was perfectly flat. It was a moment I will never forget (Figs. 18.8 and 18.9).

Only 2 days later, I was back home in the North East to continue my recovery. The day after getting home, I took a trip to town and bought a couple of tee shirts – they fitted properly (not big, baggy ones), and were yellow and white, colours I'd avoided for three decades. I remember walking down Grey Street wearing one of the shirts, with the wind blowing into me – and realizing that my arms were not crossed. Freedom!

My recovery went as smoothly as I could possibly have hoped. I barely felt any pain at all in my chest, but did struggle with a seriously aching back for a few days, which meant I had several literally sleepless nights. I was off all pain-killing medication within a couple of weeks after the operation, and back at work within 3 weeks. I didn't overdo the exercise, but took regular short walks to help me progress.

Almost 3 years to the day of the Nuss operation, I was back at London Heart Hospital to have my bars removed. Another smooth and fuss-free experience at the hands of the wonderful hospital staff, and I was back at home the next day. And the shape of my chest had improved again following bar removal, with my rib flare even less pronounced. I don't think I will ever look at my chest in the future, and not think: "Wow – what happened to the dent!"

So, is that the end of my pectus excavatum story? In one way, it's just the beginning. I've been through the journey now, and reflect on it with only great positivity. I have a tougher experience ahead, as I make that same journey with my son, Daniel. He has met Dr. Kolvekar, and, when the time is right, is hoping he can change his life beyond measure, as he changed mine…

References

1. Habelt S, Korn S, Berger A, Jozef Bielek J. Psychological distress in patients with pectus excavatum as an indication for therapy. IJCM. 2011;2(3): 295–300.
2. Ji Y, Liu W, Chen S, Xu B, Tang Y, Wang X, Yang G, Cao L. Assessment of psychosocial functioning and its risk factors in children with pectus excavatum. Health Qual Life Outcomes. 2011;9:1–8.

Index

A
Acquired chest wall deformities, 99–106
Acquired Jeune's syndrome, 102, 104, 117
Acquired pectus carinatum, 105
Acquired restrictive thoracic dystrophy
    (ARTD), 102, 104, 105
Anterior chest wall, 1, 26, 31, 36, 42, 43, 49, 71, 87,
    100, 101, 104–106, 115, 116, 119, 121, 123,
    146, 158, 161
ARTD. *See* Acquired restrictive thoracic
    dystrophy (ARTD)
Asphyxiating thoracic dystrophy (ATD), 4, 33, 92, 93,
    102, 117

C
Cardiopulmonary function, 19, 36, 87–90
Cardiovascular magnetic resonance (CMR), 28–31
Chest wall deformity(ies), 2–3, 9–11, 16, 17, 21, 25–33,
    47, 50, 61–65, 71, 75, 79–84, 90–96, 99–106,
    129–132, 134, 135, 140, 147, 153
Chest wall infection, 100
Chest wall tumor, 100, 101
Chest x-ray, 26–28, 31, 36–42, 52, 53, 155
CMR. *See* Cardiovascular magnetic resonance (CMR)
Complications, 2, 4, 15, 64, 65, 69, 74–77, 80, 82–84,
    102, 105, 106, 111–113, 115, 117, 118, 124,
    132, 138, 139, 151, 154, 158
Congenital chest wall deformity, 3, 9, 17, 71, 75
Congenital deformity, 1, 87
Conservative treatment, 138–141
Costal cartilages, 1, 7, 9, 11, 14, 25, 31, 32, 39, 62, 63,
    71, 79, 102, 105, 112, 115, 121, 138, 146

D
Dynamic compressor system (DCS), 138, 146–151,
    153–155, 158

E
Epidemiology, 7–11, 15–16

F
Failure, 17, 65, 92, 105, 109–111, 113, 124, 147, 148,
    151, 155, 159
Fat grafting, 132–135
Funnel chest, 3, 17, 88, 139
Funnel-form chest, 13

H
Haller index, 26–29, 36, 37, 41–48, 52–54, 58, 68, 80,
    90, 117, 118, 130

I
Iatrogenic deformites, 100–106
Imaging, 26–29, 31–33, 41, 42, 82, 102, 117, 131
Implants, 15, 80, 131–133, 158

J
Jeune syndrome, 4, 33, 92

L
Lung herniation, 32, 105

M
Magnetic resonance imaging (MRI), 28–33, 36, 37,
    51–53, 90, 119, 131, 138, 155
Malformation, 7, 10, 11, 35, 36, 43, 44, 52, 53, 56, 92,
    93, 100, 101, 105, 122, 143
Mammoplasty, 131–132
Minimally invasive, 2, 3, 14, 64, 65, 71–77, 79, 88, 109,
    112, 113, 120, 138, 161
MRI. *See* Magnetic resonance imaging (MRI)
Multi-modal analgesia, 84

N
Non-operative treatment, 146, 151, 158
Non-steroidal anti-inflammatory drugs, 79, 84

© Springer International Publishing Switzerland 2016
S.K. Kolvekar, H.K. Pilegaard (eds.), *Chest Wall Deformities and Corrective Procedures*,
DOI 10.1007/978-3-319-23968-2